MAYO CLINIC

The Essential Diabetes Book

SECOND EDITION

MAYO CLINIC

Medical Editor
M. Regina Castro, M.D.

Managing Editor
Jennifer L. Duesterhoeft

Editorial Director
Paula Marlow Limbeck

Product Manager
Christopher C. Frye

Creative Director
Daniel W. Brevick

Art Director
Richard A. Resnick

Illustrators
Tristan Cummings, Kent McDaniel

Research Librarians
Anthony J. Cook, Amanda K. Golden, Deirdre A. Herman, Erika A. Riggin

Proofreaders
Miranda M. Attlesey, Donna L. Hanson, Julie M. Maas

Indexer
Steve Rath

Administrative Assistant
Beverly J. Steele

Contributing Editors
Donald D. Hensrud, M.D., Nancy M. Klobassa-Davidson, R.N., Seema Kumar, M.D., Jennifer K. Nelson, R.D., L.D., Paula Ricke, Pankaj Shah, M.D., Steven A. Smith, M.D., Sara E. Weigel, R.D., L.D.

TIME HOME ENTERTAINMENT INC.

President and Publisher
Jim Childs

Vice President, Brand & Digital Strategy
Steven Sandonato

Vice President, Finance
Vandana Patel

Executive Director, Marketing Services
Carol Pittard

Executive Director, Retail & Special Sales
Tom Mifsud

Executive Publishing Director
Joy Butts

Publishing Director
Megan Pearlman

Director, Bookazine Development & Marketing
Laura Adam

Associate General Counsel
Helen Wan

OXMOOR HOUSE

Vice President, Brand Publishing
Laura Sappington

Editorial Director
Leah McLaughlin

Creative Director
Felicity Keane

Senior Brand Manager
Nina Fleishman

Managing Editor
Elizabeth Tyler Austin

Assistant Managing Editor
Jeanne de Lathouder

MAYO CLINIC THE ESSENTIAL DIABETES BOOK

Art Director
Christopher Rhoads

Senior Production Manager
Greg A. Amason

Associate Production Manager
Amy Mangus

Special thanks to: Katherine Barnet, Jeremy Biloon, Susan Chodakiewicz, Rose Cirrincione, Jacqueline Fitzgerald, Christine Font, Jenna Goldberg, Hillary Hirsch, David Kahn, Mona Li, Amy Mangus, Amy Migliaccio, Nina Mistry, Dave Rozzelle, Ricardo Santiago, Adriana Tierno, Vanessa Wu

Published by Time Home Entertainment Inc.

135 W. 50th St. • New York, NY 10020

ISBN-13: 978-0-8487-4339-0

ISBN-10: 0-8487-4339-3

Library of Congress Control Number: 2014933598

Second Edition

Printed in the United States of America

Mayo Clinic The Essential Diabetes Book is intended to supplement the advice of your personal physician, whom you should consult regarding individual medical conditions. MAYO, MAYO CLINIC and the Mayo triple-shield logo are marks of Mayo Foundation for Medical Education and Research.

We welcome your comments and suggestions about Time Home Entertainment Books. Please write to us at Time Home Entertainment Books, Attention: Book Editors, P.O. Box 11016, Des Moines, IA 50336-1016

If you would like to order any of our hardcover Collector's Edition books, please call us at 800-327-6388, Monday through Friday, 7 a.m. to 8 p.m., or Saturday, 7 a.m. to 6 p.m., Central time.

For bulk sales to employers, member groups and health-related companies, contact Mayo Clinic Health Solutions, 200 First St. SW, Rochester, MN 55905, or send an email to *SpecialSalesMayoBooks@Mayo.edu.*

We do not endorse any company or product.

Cover design by Christopher Rhoads

Photo credits:
There is no correlation between the individuals portrayed and the conditions or subjects being discussed.

Introduction

It's rare to meet someone who doesn't aspire to live a long and healthy life. Often, our desire for longevity is motivated by goals — a desire to achieve something — be it a personal or professional accomplishment. It might be a desire to raise a family, be a teacher, be a professional athlete or simply be a part of your grandchildren's lives.

Although you may have great genes on your side, none of us is guaranteed health and longevity. Today, more than ever, you have to assume responsibility for your future and play an active role in protecting your health. This is especially true for people with, or at risk of, diabetes.

The good news is that despite the challenges you may be facing, there are multiple opportunities to improve and protect your health. Our goal — mine and those of the other contributors to this book — is to help you identify and act upon those opportunities. And in encouraging this action, we hope to keep you on the path to good health.

Diabetes is serious — and increasingly common. But you can learn how to successfully control the disease and lead a healthy and productive life. In this book, we provide you key steps to living well with diabetes. This includes essential advice on how to monitor your blood sugar, how to eat better, how to become more physically active, how to lose weight and maintain a healthy weight, and how to get the most from your medications.

If you have a child with diabetes, you'll also learn practical tips, from recognizing key signs and symptoms, to involving your child in diabetes care, to dealing with emotional issues.

Read through this book with a positive attitude. The right attitude will not only help you add years to your life but also allow you to enjoy them.

M. Regina Castro, M.D.
Medical Editor

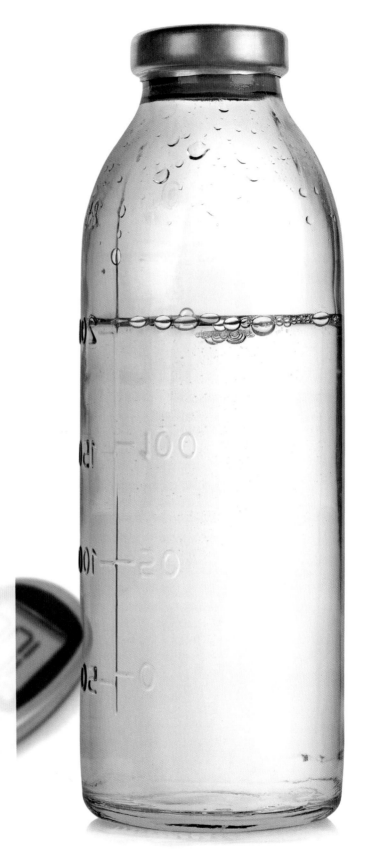

Table of Contents

Chapter 1 **Understanding Diabetes** **8**

What is diabetes? 10

The different types 11

Signs and symptoms 15

Are you at risk? 17

Tests to detect diabetes 20

Diabetes dangers 21

Medical emergencies 21

Long-term complications 26

Chapter 2 **Monitoring Your Blood Sugar** **30**

How often and when to test 32

What you'll need 33

Performing the test 35

Advances in monitoring tools 36

Recording your results 38

Keeping within your range 40

Troubleshooting problems 41

When test results signal a problem 46

Avoiding the highs and lows 46

Overcoming barriers 49

Chapter 3 **Developing a Healthy-Eating Plan** **50**

Debunking the diabetes 'diet' 52

What's healthy eating? 52

Plan your meals 57

Watch your serving sizes 58

Size up your plate 60

Read food labels 61

Consider carb counting 62

The scoop on sugar 64

Using exchange lists 65

Keeping motivated 67

Recipes for good health 68

Chapter 4 **Achieving a Healthy Weight** **84**

Do you need to lose weight? 86

Assess your readiness 88

Set realistic goals 92

Simple first steps 94

The Mayo Clinic Healthy Weight Pyramid 95

Energy density: Eat more and lose weight 98

Keeping a food record 101

What are your eating triggers? 103

What's your meal routine? 104
Adapting recipes 106
Be a smart shopper 107
Bumps in the road: Overcoming setbacks 109

Chapter 5   **Getting More Active** **112**
Physical activity vs. exercise 114
Fitness is essential to your health 115
Create a personal fitness plan 117
Tackle your exercise barriers 120
Aerobic exercise 122
Walking to better health 124
Staying hydrated 128
How much exercise? 129
Stretching exercises 130
Strengthening exercises 132
Avoiding injury 135
Exercise and regular monitoring 136
Getting and staying motivated 137
Fitness for kids 140

Chapter 6   **Medical Treatment** **142**
Insulin therapy 144
How to inject insulin 149
Avoiding insulin problems 153
Insulin pumps 154
Oral diabetes medications 156
Oral drug combinations 162
Oral drugs and insulin 162
Injectable drugs 164
Kidney dialysis 165
Kidney transplant 167
Other transplant procedures 167

Chapter 7   **Staying Healthy** **170**
Yearly checkups 173
Important tests you should have 174
Caring for your eyes 179
Caring for your feet 180
Caring for your teeth 183
Getting vaccinated 184
Managing stress 184
Preparing for pregnancy 190
Understanding menstruation and diabetes 195
Dealing with menopause 195
Living with erectile dysfunction 196

Chapter 8   **If Your Child Has Diabetes**. **200**

Type 1 diabetes. 203
Type 2 diabetes. 205
Caring for medical needs. 208
Emotional and social issues. 210
Good habits for staying healthy 212
Surviving sick days 215

Additional Resources. **218**

Index. **220**

Chapter 1
Understanding Diabetes

What is diabetes? 10

The different types 11

Signs and symptoms 15

Are you at risk? 17

Tests to detect diabetes 20

Diabetes dangers 21

Medical emergencies 21

Long-term complications 26

A visit with Dr. Regina Castro

"This threat to our general health is significant enough that for the first time in history, younger generations may not enjoy the long lives that we have come to expect."

We seem to be involved in a losing fight. The number of individuals diagnosed with diabetes, particularly type 2 diabetes mellitus, continues to rise.

In addition, we're seeing more young people with type 2 diabetes — many children and adolescents — as well as people of varied ethnic backgrounds and all forms of economic status. This threat to our general health is significant enough that for the first time in history, younger generations may not enjoy the long lives that we have come to expect.

What's driving this epidemic? Have our genes changed dramatically? The answer is NO! What has changed is the way we lead our lives. Meals are often not prepared at home but eaten on the run, high in fat and calories, and low in fruits and vegetables. We've become less physically active, both at work and in our leisure time, and as a result most of us are either overweight or obese. The impact of excess weight on health is astounding. It increases the risk of diabetes and predisposes people to many other health problems, including some types of cancer.

It's clear that we can't solve this problem in doctors' offices — we've tried and failed. Physicians and patients alike have to extend their focus beyond the confines of the doctor's office, clinic or hospital. As a general population, we have to focus on the decisions we make every day that affect our health, whether it's at home, work or school. This requires change, and change is often hard.

When you face a big challenge, you want the best people on your side. In this publication, we've recruited the help of experts who play important roles in the care of people with diabetes of all ages. Their advice will help you understand diabetes and recognize how sometimes small, everyday decisions can help you control your disease and protect your health. When you promote healthy-eating habits and regular

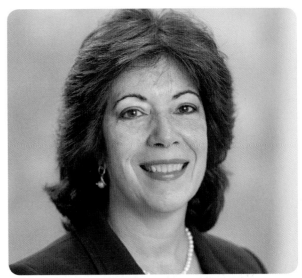

M. Regina Castro, M.D.
Endocrinology

© MFMER

physical activity, your efforts can also help protect the health of those around you, regardless of their ages.

As much as I believe in the importance of these changes, I know how challenging making them can be. By reading this essential guide, you've taken a first step in empowering yourself toward a healthier lifestyle. The information here will arm you with knowledge, but in order for this knowledge to help you, it needs to be put into action. Identifying the obstacles that keep you from eating healthy, being more physically active and taking better care of yourself are the first steps. Then recruit individuals who can help you overcome those obstacles. It can be a dietitian helping you find ways to improve your eating habits. It can be a co-worker encouraging you to walk during your work break. It can be your employer promoting healthier food choices at work. And yes, it should include your health care provider.

In our constantly changing environment, your role in protecting your health is more important than ever. We hope you find the information available here a helpful tool at fulfilling that role.

Perhaps your doctor recently broke the news that you have diabetes. Or you've learned that you're at risk of getting the disease. You're worried — afraid of what diabetes will do to you. Will you have to eat tasteless food that has no sugar? Will you have to give yourself daily shots of insulin? Will you eventually face an amputation? Will your diabetes kill you?

For the majority of individuals with diabetes, the answer to these questions is no. Researchers have learned a great deal about how to diagnose diabetes early and how to control it. Because of these advances, you can live well and not suffer serious complications if you follow your doctor's advice regarding eating, exercise, blood sugar (glucose) monitoring and, when necessary, use of medications.

You can enjoy an active and healthy life despite having diabetes, but you have to be willing to do your part.

What is diabetes?

The term *diabetes* refers to a group of diseases that affect the way your body uses blood glucose, commonly called blood sugar. Glucose is vital to your health because it's the main source of energy for the cells that make up your muscles and tissues. It's your body's main source of fuel.

If you have diabetes — no matter what type — it means you have too much glucose in your blood, although the reasons why may differ. And too much glucose can lead to serious problems.

To understand diabetes, it helps to understand how your body normally processes blood glucose.

Processing of blood glucose

Blood glucose comes from two major sources: the food you eat and your liver. During digestion, glucose is absorbed into your bloodstream. Normally, it then enters your body's cells, aided by the action of insulin. The hormone insulin comes from your pancreas. When you eat, your pancreas secretes insulin into your bloodstream.

As insulin circulates, it acts like a key, unlocking microscopic doors that allow glucose to enter your cells. In this way, insulin lowers the amount of glucose in your bloodstream and prevents it from reaching high levels.

As your blood glucose level drops, so does the secretion of insulin from your pancreas. Your liver acts as a glucose storage and manufacturing center. When the level of insulin in your blood is high, such as after a meal, your liver stores extra glucose as glycogen in case your cells need it later.

Normal metabolism

Extra glucose is stored in the liver.

Glucose is broken down from the sugar in food.

Insulin leaves the pancreas and enters the bloodstream.

Insulin escorts and allows glucose into your cells, where it's needed for energy. Without insulin, glucose remains "locked" outside of the cells.

© MFMER

When your insulin levels are low, for example, when you haven't eaten in a while, your liver releases the stored glucose into your bloodstream to keep your blood sugar level within a normal range.

When you have diabetes

If you have diabetes, this process doesn't work properly. Instead of being transported into your cells, excess glucose builds up in your bloodstream, and eventually some of it is excreted in your urine. This usually occurs when your pancreas produces little or no insulin, or your cells don't respond properly to insulin, or for both reasons.

The medical term for this condition is diabetes mellitus (MEL-lih-tuhs). *Mellitus* is a Latin word meaning "honey sweet," referring to the excess sugar in your blood and urine.

Another form of diabetes, called diabetes insipidus (in-SIP-uh-dus), is a rare condition in which the kidneys are unable to conserve water, leading to increased urination and excessive thirst. Rather than an insulin problem, diabetes insipidus results from a different hormone disorder.

In this book, the term *diabetes* refers only to diabetes mellitus.

The different types

People often think of diabetes as one disease. But glucose can accumulate in your blood for various reasons, resulting in different types of diabetes. The two most common forms are type 1 and type 2.

Type 1

Type 1 diabetes develops when your pancreas makes little if any insulin. Without insulin circulating in your bloodstream, glucose can't get into your cells, so it remains in your blood.

Type 1 diabetes used to be called insulin-dependent diabetes and juvenile diabetes. That's because

? If I have a close relative with type 1 diabetes, what are my chances of getting the disease?

For reasons that aren't well-understood, your risk of developing diabetes varies. Note in the chart at right that family history — which includes both learned behavior and genetics — along with lifestyle, seems to play a larger role in the development of type 2 diabetes than type 1. Many people with type 1 diabetes have no known family history.

How does family history affect your risk of diabetes?

Type 1		Type 2	
Relative with diabetes	Your estimated risk	Relative with diabetes	Your estimated risk
Mother	1 to 5%	Mother	5 to 20%
Father	5 to 15%	Father	5 to 20%
Both parents	1 to 25%	Both parents	25 to 50%
Brother/sister	5 to 10%	Brother/sister	25 to 50%
Identical twin	25 to 50%	Identical twin	60 to 75%

Based on a review of recent medical journal articles and textbooks

Are you at risk of type 2 diabetes?

 Place a check mark in any of the boxes below that apply to you. The more boxes that you check, the higher your risk of type 2 diabetes.

❑ Parent, brother or sister with type 2 diabetes
❑ Overweight
❑ Carry excess weight around waist or upper body (apple shape) rather than hips and thighs (pear shape)
❑ Not physically active — get little or no exercise
❑ Older than age 45
❑ Black American, Hispanic-American, American Indian, Alaska Native, Asian-American or Pacific Islander
❑ Gave birth to a baby who weighed more than 9 pounds
❑ Developed diabetes when pregnant (gestational diabetes)

the disease most often develops when you're a child or a teen, and daily insulin shots are needed to make up for the insulin your body doesn't produce.

However, the names *insulin-dependent diabetes* and *juvenile diabetes* aren't entirely accurate. Although less common, adults also can develop type 1 diabetes. And the use of insulin isn't limited to people with type 1 disease. People with other forms of diabetes also may need insulin.

Type 1 diabetes is an autoimmune disease, meaning that your own immune system is the culprit. Similar to how it attacks invading viruses or bacteria, your body's infection-fighting system attacks your pancreas, zeroing in on your beta cells, which produce insulin. Researchers aren't certain what causes your immune system to fight your own body, but they believe genetic factors, exposure to certain viruses and diet may be involved.

The attacks can dramatically reduce — even entirely wipe out — the insulin-making capacity of your pancreas. Between 5 and 10 percent of people with diabetes have type 1, with the disease occurring almost equally among males and females.

The process leading to type 1 diabetes can occur slowly, so the disease may go undetected for several months or possibly longer. More often, though, signs and symptoms come on quickly, commonly following an illness.

Type 2

Type 2 diabetes is by far the most common form of the disease. Ninety to 95 percent of people older than age 20 who have diabetes have type 2. Like type 1 diabetes, type 2 used to be called by other names: noninsulin-dependent diabetes and adult-onset diabetes. These names reflect that many people with type 2 diabetes don't need insulin shots and that the disease usually develops in adults.

As with type 1, these names aren't entirely accurate. That's because children and teenagers, as well as adults, can develop type 2 disease. In fact, the incidence of type 2 diabetes in children and adolescents is increasing. In addition, many people with type 2 diabetes need insulin to control their blood glucose.

Unlike type 1, type 2 diabetes isn't an autoimmune disease. With type 2 diabetes, your pancreas makes insulin, but your cells become resistant to it. So insulin can't help move glucose into your cells. As a result, most of the glucose stays in your bloodstream and accumulates. Exactly why the cells become resistant to insulin is uncertain, although excess weight and fatty tissue seem to be important factors. Most people who develop type 2 diabetes are overweight.

Some people with type 2 diabetes eventually require insulin shots. That's because the pancreas may not produce enough insulin, or it may lose its ability to make insulin. Like people with type 1 diabetes, people with type 2 disease may become dependent on insulin.

Other types

Type 1 and type 2 are the most common forms of diabetes, and therefore they receive the most attention. The disease, however, can present itself in other forms.

Gestational

Gestational diabetes is the name for diabetes that develops during pregnancy. Diabetes can develop temporarily when hormones secreted during pregnancy increase your body's resistance to insulin. This happens in about 5 percent of pregnant women in the United States, although estimates vary.

Gestational diabetes typically develops during the second half of pregnancy — especially in the third trimester — and goes away after the baby is born. But about half of all women who experience gestational diabetes develop type 2 diabetes later in life.

Most pregnant women are screened for gestational diabetes to catch the condition early. If you develop gestational diabetes, being aware of your condition and controlling your blood glucose level throughout your pregnancy can reduce complications for you and your baby.

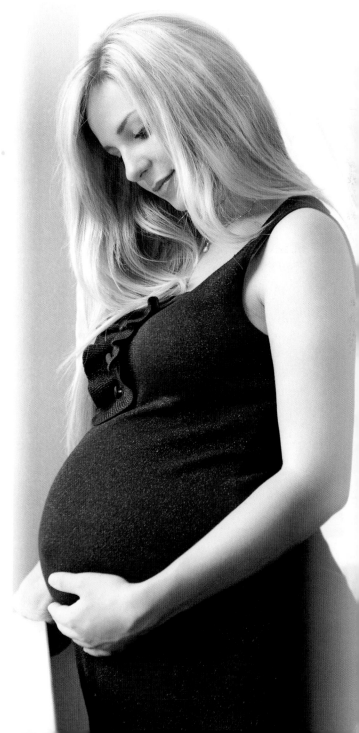

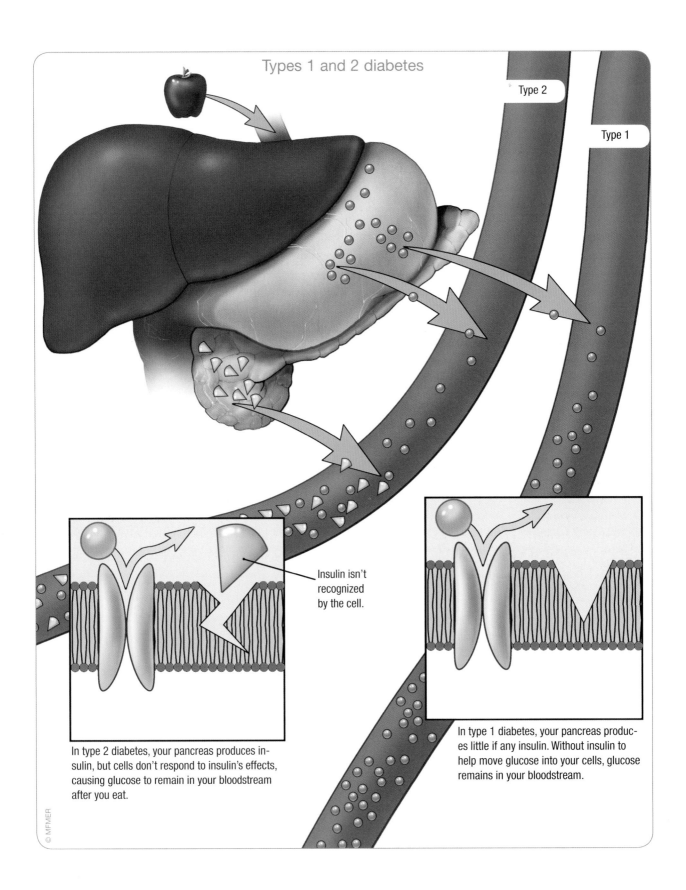

Types 1 and 2 diabetes

Type 2

Type 1

Insulin isn't recognized by the cell.

In type 2 diabetes, your pancreas produces insulin, but cells don't respond to insulin's effects, causing glucose to remain in your bloodstream after you eat.

In type 1 diabetes, your pancreas produces little if any insulin. Without insulin to help move glucose into your cells, glucose remains in your bloodstream.

© MFMER

LADA and MODY

Latent autoimmune diabetes of adults (LADA) is a form of type 1 diabetes that develops slowly over many years. LADA is uncommon, but it can be mistaken for type 2 diabetes.

Maturity-onset diabetes of youth (MODY) is an uncommon form of type 2 diabetes, caused by a defect in a single gene. MODY generally affects young people with a family history of the condition.

Other causes

A small number of diagnosed cases of diabetes result from conditions or medications that can interfere with the production of insulin or its action. They include inflammation of the pancreas (pancreatitis), pancreas removal, adrenal or pituitary gland disorders, rare genetic defects, infection, malnutrition, and medications used to treat another disease.

Diabetes warning signs

Whether you have type 1 or type 2 diabetes, the classic signs and symptoms are:
- Excessive thirst
- Increased urination

Other signs and symptoms may include:
- Constant hunger
- Flu-like symptoms, including weakness and fatigue
- Unexplained weight loss
- Blurred vision
- Slow-healing cuts or bruises
- Tingling or loss of feeling in hands and feet
- Recurring bladder or vaginal infections
- Recurring infections of gums or skin

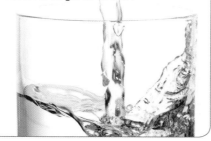

Signs and symptoms

Like many people, you may have been shocked to learn that you have diabetes because you weren't experiencing any symptoms. You felt fine. Often there are no early symptoms.

This is especially true with type 2 diabetes. Lack of symptoms and the slow emergence of the disease are the main reasons type 2 diabetes often goes undetected for years. When symptoms do develop from persistently high blood glucose, they vary.

Two classic symptoms that occur in most people with the disease are increased thirst and a frequent need to urinate.

Excessive thirst and increased urination

When you have high levels of glucose in your blood, it overwhelms your kidneys' filtering system. Your kidneys can't resorb all of the excess sugar, and it's excreted into your urine with fluids drawn from your tissues. This process leads to more frequent urination. As a result, you feel dehydrated. To replace the fluids being drawn out, you're almost constantly drinking water or other beverages.

Flu-like feeling

Symptoms of diabetes, such as fatigue, weakness and loss of appetite, can mimic a viral illness. That's because when you have diabetes and it's not well-controlled, the process of using glucose for energy is impaired, affecting your body's function.

Weight loss or gain

Some people, especially those with type 1 diabetes, lose weight before diagnosis. That's because glucose lost through urination leads to calorie loss. More stored fat is used for energy, and muscle tissues may not get enough glucose to generate growth. The weight loss might not be noticeable in people with type 2 diabetes because they tend to be overweight. But in most people with type 2 and some people with type 1, diabetes develops after a period of weight gain. Excess weight worsens insulin resistance, leading to an increase in blood sugar levels.

Blurred vision

Excessive glucose in your blood draws the fluid out of the lenses in your eyes, causing them to thin and affecting their ability to focus. Lowering your blood sugar helps restore fluid to your lenses. Your vision may remain blurry for a while as your lenses adjust to the restoration of fluid. But in time vision typically improves. High blood glucose can also cause the formation of tiny blood vessels in your eyes that can bleed. The blood vessels themselves don't produce symptoms, but bleeding from the vessels can cause dark spots, flashing lights, rings around lights and even blindness.

Because diabetes-related eye changes often don't produce symptoms, it's important that you see an eye specialist (ophthalmologist or optometrist) regularly. By dilating your pupils, an eye specialist is able to examine the blood vessels in each retina.

Slow-healing sores or frequent infections

High levels of blood glucose block your body's natural healing process and its ability to fight off infections. For women, bladder and vaginal infections are especially common.

Tingling feet and hands

Too much glucose in your blood can damage your nerves, which are nourished by your blood. Nerve damage can produce a number of symptoms. The most common are a tingling feeling and a loss of sensation that occurs mainly in your feet and hands. This results from damage to your sensory nerves. You may also experience pain in your extremities — legs, feet, arms and hands — including burning pain.

Red, swollen and tender gums

Diabetes can also weaken your mouth's ability to fight germs. This increases the risk of infection in your gums and the bones that help hold your teeth in place. Signs and symptoms of gum disease include:

▶ Gums that have pulled away from your teeth, exposing more of your teeth or even part of the root
▶ Sores or pockets of pus in your gums
▶ Permanent teeth becoming loose
▶ Changes in the fit of your dentures

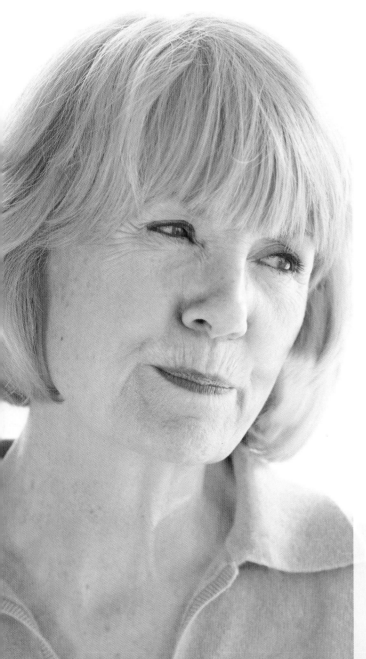

Are you at risk?

Perhaps you've heard one of the common myths about diabetes — that it comes from eating too much sugar. That's not true. Researchers don't fully understand why some people develop the disease and others don't. It's clear, though, that your lifestyle and certain health conditions can increase your risk.

Family history

Your chance of developing either type 1 or type 2 diabetes increases if someone in your immediate family has the disease, whether that person is a parent, brother or sister (see the chart on page 12). Genetics plays a role in the disease, but exactly how certain genes may cause diabetes is unknown. Scientists are studying genes that may be linked to diabetes, but tests are still under development and not available for routine clinical use.

Although people who develop diabetes may have inherited a tendency toward the disease, some type of environmental factor usually triggers this tendency.

Weight

Being overweight or obese is one of the most common risk factors for type 2 diabetes. More than 80 percent of people with type 2 diabetes are overweight or obese. The more fatty tissue you have, the more resistant your muscle and tissue cells become to your own insulin. This is especially true if your excess weight is concentrated around your abdomen and your body is an apple shape rather than a pear shape, in which the weight is mostly on the hips and thighs.

Many people with diabetes who are overweight can improve their blood glucose levels simply by losing weight. Even a small weight loss can have beneficial effects, reducing blood sugar or allowing diabetes medications to work better.

Inactivity

The less active you are, the greater your risk of type 2 diabetes. Physical activity helps you control your weight, uses up sugar as energy, makes your cells more sensitive to insulin, increases blood flow and improves circulation. Exercise also helps build muscle mass. That's

Estimated percentage of U.S. adults with diabetes by race and ethnicity

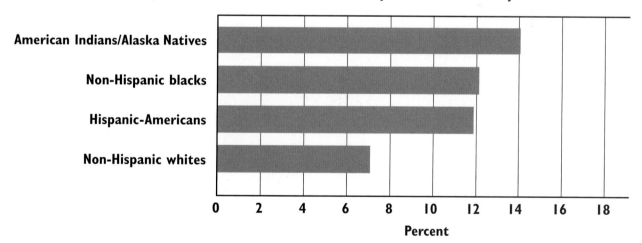

It's estimated that about 7 percent of non-Hispanic white adults (age 20 and older) have type 1 or type 2 diabetes. But the percentage of adults with diabetes is higher in other groups, affecting almost 14 percent of American Indians and Alaska Natives, more than 12 percent of non-Hispanic blacks, and almost 12 percent of Hispanic-Americans.
Adapted from Centers for Disease Control and Prevention, 2011

Estimated percentage of U.S. adults with diabetes by age group

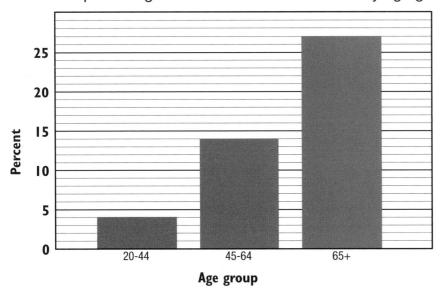

It's estimated that nearly 4 percent of adults ages 20 to 44, 14 percent of adults ages 45 to 64, and 27 percent of adults age 65 and older have type 1 or 2 diabetes.

Adapted from National Institute of Diabetes and Digestive and Kidney Diseases, 2011

important because most of the glucose in your blood is absorbed by your muscles and burned as energy.

Age

Your risk of type 2 diabetes increases as you grow older, especially after age 45. At least 1 in 5 Americans age 65 and older has diabetes. Part of the reason is that as people grow older they tend to become less physically active, and they gradually lose muscle mass and gain weight.

Recent years, however, have shown a dramatic rise in type 2 diabetes among people in their 30s and 40s. In addition, more children and teenagers are being diagnosed with type 2 diabetes.

Race and ethnicity

About 8 percent of the U.S. population has diabetes. Although it's unclear why, people of certain races are more likely to develop diabetes than are others.

Type 1 diabetes is more common in white Americans than in black Americans, Hispanic-Americans, or other ethnic groups or races. However, if you're a black American or Hispanic-American, you're about 1.5 times more likely to have type 2 diabetes than is someone who's white.

If you're an American Indian or Alaska Native, your risk of type 2 diabetes more than doubles compared with whites. Asian-Americans and Pacific Islanders also have a higher risk of type 2 diabetes than do white Americans.

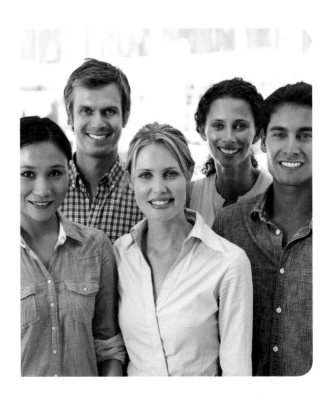

Metabolic syndrome and diabetes

Metabolic syndrome (also called insulin resistance syndrome) is a cluster of metabolic disorders that makes you more likely to develop type 2 diabetes, heart disease and stroke. You may have metabolic syndrome if you have three or more of the following risk factors:

▶ **Abdominal obesity.** More than a 35-inch waist for women and more than a 40-inch waist for men*

▶ **Triglycerides.** A level of 150 milligrams per deciliter (mg/dL) of blood or above, or drug treatment for high triglycerides

▶ **High-density lipoprotein cholesterol, the 'good' kind.** Lower than 50 mg/dL for women and lower than 40 mg/dL for men, or drug treatment for low HDL

▶ **Blood pressure.** Top number (systolic) of 130 mm Hg or above or bottom number (diastolic) of 85 mm Hg or above, or drug treatment for high blood pressure

▶ **Fasting blood glucose.** A level of 100 mg/dL or higher, or drug treatment for high blood glucose

If you think that you have metabolic syndrome, talk with your doctor about tests that can help determine this. A balanced diet, healthy weight and increasing your level of physical activity can help combat metabolic syndrome and play a role in preventing diabetes and other serious diseases.

*For Asian-Americans: More than a 31-inch waist for women and more than a 35-inch waist for men
Adapted from American Heart Association and National Heart, Lung, and Blood Institute, 2005

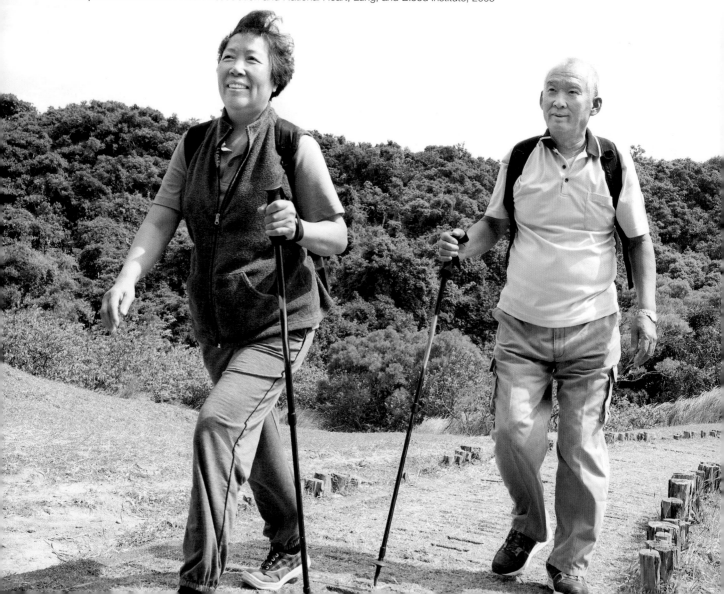

Tests to detect diabetes

Many people learn they have diabetes through blood tests done for another condition or as part of a physical exam. Sometimes, though, a doctor may test specifically for diabetes if he or she suspects the disease, based on symptoms or risk factors.

An international committee of experts from the American Diabetes Association, the European Association for the Study of Diabetes and the International Diabetes Federation recommends that type 1 and type 2 diabetes testing include four tests.

Glycated hemoglobin (A1C) test

This blood test indicates your average blood sugar level for the past two to three months. It works by measuring the percentage of blood sugar attached to hemoglobin, the oxygen-carrying protein in red blood cells. The higher your blood sugar levels, the more hemoglobin you'll have with sugar attached. An A1C level of 6.5 percent or higher on two separate tests indicates you have diabetes. See page 174 for more information on this test.

If the A1C test isn't available, or if you have certain conditions that can make the A1C test inaccurate — such as if you're pregnant or you have an uncommon form of hemoglobin — your doctor may use other tests.

Random blood glucose test

This test may be a part of the routine blood work done during a physical exam. Using a needle inserted into a vein, blood is drawn for a variety of laboratory tests. This is done without any special preparation on your part, such as an overnight fast.

Even if you've recently eaten before the test and your blood glucose is at its peak, the level shouldn't be above 200 milligrams of glucose per deciliter of blood (mg/dL). If it is, and if you're experiencing signs and symptoms of diabetes, you can expect a diagnosis of diabetes.

Fasting blood glucose test

The amount of glucose in your blood naturally fluctuates, but within a narrow range. Your blood glucose level is typically highest after a meal and lowest after an overnight fast. The preferred way to test your blood glucose is after you've fasted overnight or for at least eight hours.

Blood is drawn from a vein and sent to a lab for evaluation. A fasting blood sugar level between 70 and 99 mg/dL is normal. If the results on two separate tests show a level between 100 and 125 mg/dL, you have what's known as prediabetes.

Prediabetes shouldn't be taken lightly. It's a sign that you're at high risk of developing diabetes and that you should see your doctor regularly and take steps to control your glucose.

What the results mean

An international committee of diabetes experts recommends the A1C test for prediabetes and diabetes testing. If the A1C test isn't available, the fasting blood glucose test is another option.

A1C test results	Indicates
Less than 5.7%	Normal
Between 5.7 and 6.4%	Prediabetes*
6.5% or higher on 2 separate tests	Diabetes

Fasting blood glucose test results	Indicates
Under 100 mg/dL†	Normal
100 to 125 mg/dL	Prediabetes
126 mg/dL or higher on 2 separate tests	Diabetes

*Prediabetes means that you're at high risk of developing diabetes.
†milligrams of glucose per deciliter of blood
Adapted from American Diabetes Association, 2012

> **?** Is the risk of death after a heart attack higher in people with diabetes than in people who don't have diabetes?
>
> **Yes.** People with diabetes are more likely to have high blood pressure and high cholesterol, which increase damage to the arteries that supply oxygen to the heart (coronary arteries), causing a more severe attack. In addition, people with diabetes are less likely to experience typical symptoms of a heart attack, so they may not seek medical attention as quickly.

Readings of 126 mg/dL or higher on two separate tests indicate diabetes. If your blood glucose is above 200 mg/dL, with symptoms of diabetes, a second test may not be necessary to reach the diagnosis.

Oral glucose tolerance test

This test is not commonly used today because other tests are less expensive and easier to administer.

An oral glucose tolerance test requires that you visit a lab or your doctor's office after at least an eight-hour fast. There you drink about 8 ounces of a sweet liquid that contains a lot of sugar — about 75 grams. Your blood glucose is measured before you drink the liquid, after one hour and again after two hours.

Doctors sometimes use a modified version of this test to check pregnant women for gestational diabetes.

Diabetes dangers

Diabetes is often easy to ignore, especially in the early stages. You're feeling fine. Your body seems to be working well. No symptoms. No problem. Right? Not even close.

While you're doing nothing, the excess glucose in your blood is eroding the very fabric of your body, threatening major organs, including your heart,

nerves, eyes and kidneys. You may not feel the effects right away, but eventually you will.

Compared with people who don't have diabetes, when you have diabetes you're two times more likely to suffer a heart attack, stroke and death from cardiovascular disease. Among adults in the United States, diabetes is the leading cause of:

- New cases of blindness in people ages 20 to 74
- Limb amputation
- Kidney failure

Researchers are making great progress in understanding what triggers complications of diabetes and how to manage or prevent them. Several studies show that if you keep your blood glucose close to normal, you can dramatically reduce your risks of complications.

And it's never too late to start. As soon as you begin managing your glucose level, you may slow the progression of complications and reduce your chances of developing more health problems.

Medical emergencies

Medical emergencies require immediate attention. If you experience any of the following signs or symptoms, get medical help right away.

Low blood sugar (hypoglycemia)

Low blood glucose — a level below 70 mg/dL — is called hypoglycemia (hi-po-gli-SEE-mee-uh). This condition basically results from too much insulin and too little glucose in your blood. If your blood glucose level drops too low — for example, below 50 mg/dL — this could result in confusion, seizures or a loss of consciousness, a condition sometimes called insulin shock or coma.

Hypoglycemia, also called an insulin reaction, is most common among people taking insulin. It can also occur in people taking oral medications that enhance the release of insulin. Your blood glucose level can drop for many reasons, such as:

- Skipping or delaying a meal
- Eating too few carbohydrates
- Exercising longer or more strenuously than normal
- Having too much insulin from not adjusting your medication when you experience changes in your blood glucose

What are the signs and symptoms?

Signs and symptoms of hypoglycemia vary, depending on how low your blood glucose level drops.

Early signs and symptoms:

- Sweating
- Nervousness
- Weakness
- Irritability
- Shakiness
- Headache
- Hunger
- Nausea
- Visual disturbances
- Fast heartbeat
- Dizziness
- Cold, clammy skin

Later warning signs (typically occur with a blood glucose level below 40 mg/dL):

- Slurred speech
- Drunken-like behavior
- Drowsiness
- Confusion

Emergency signs:

- Convulsions
- Unconsciousness (coma), which can be fatal

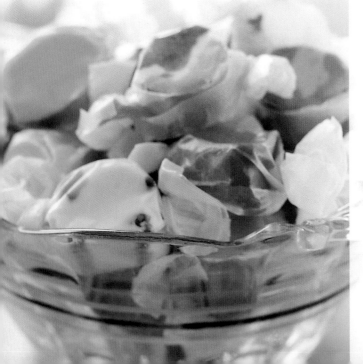

? Can you miss the early warning signs of hypoglycemia?

Some people who have had diabetes for many years don't experience early signs and symptoms of low blood glucose, such as shakiness or nervousness. That's because chemical changes from long-standing diabetes may mask the symptoms or keep them from occurring. With this condition, called hypoglycemia unawareness, you may not realize your blood glucose is low until later signs and symptoms, such as confusion or slurred speech, set in. If you're concerned about hypoglycemia unawareness, work with your health care team to identify circumstances that put you at risk of hypoglycemia and discuss ways to help prevent it.

What should you do?

As soon as you suspect that your blood glucose is low, check your glucose level. If it's below 70 mg/dL, eat or drink something that will raise your level quickly. Good examples of fast glucose-elevating solutions include:

- Hard candy, equal to about five Life Savers
- A regular (not diet) soft drink
- Half a cup of fruit juice
- Glucose tablets (nonprescription pills made especially for treating low blood glucose)

If after 15 minutes you continue to experience symptoms, repeat the treatment. If they still don't go away, contact your doctor or call for emergency assistance.

If you lose consciousness or for some other reason can't swallow, you'll need an injection of glucagon, a fast-acting hormone that stimulates the release of glucose into your blood. Teach your close friends and family members how to give you the shot in case of an emergency. Also tell them to call 911 or a local emergency number if you don't regain consciousness quickly.

A glucagon emergency kit includes the medication and a syringe. The shot is easy to administer and is generally given in an arm, buttock, thigh or the abdomen. The medication starts to act in about five minutes. If you take insulin, you should have a glucagon kit with or near you at all times. Many people have several kits and keep one in each of their vehicles, at home, at work, and in a purse or sports bag.

High blood sugar (hyperglycemia)

When your blood glucose reaches a dangerously high level, your blood actually becomes thick and syrupy. This condition, called hyperglycemic hyperosmolar (hi-pur-oz-MOE-lur) state, may occur when your blood glucose level gets over 600 mg/dL.

Your cells can't absorb this much glucose, so the glucose passes from your blood into your urine. This triggers a filtering process that draws tremendous amounts of fluid from your body and results in dehydration, a condition caused by too much water loss.

Hyperglycemic hyperosmolar state (HHS) is most common in people with type 2 diabetes, especially people who don't monitor their blood glucose or who don't know they have diabetes. It can occur in people with diabetes who are taking high-dose steroids or drugs that increase urination.

It also may be brought on by an infection (such as a urinary tract infection or pneumonia), illness, stress, drinking too much alcohol or drug abuse. Older adults with diabetes who don't get enough fluids also are at risk of HHS.

What are the signs and symptoms?

Signs and symptoms of HHS include:

- Excessive thirst
- Leg cramps
- Dry mouth
- Rapid pulse
- Frequent urination
- Seizures
- Dehydration
- Confusion
- Weakness
- Coma

What should you do?

Check your blood glucose level. If it's more than 350 mg/dL, call your doctor for advice. If it's 500 mg/dL or higher, see a doctor immediately. This is an emergency situation. Have someone else drive you to the emergency department. Don't drive yourself.

Emergency treatment can correct the problem within hours. You'll likely receive intravenous fluids to restore water to your tissues, and short-acting insulin to help your tissue cells absorb glucose. Without prompt treatment, the condition can be fatal.

High ketones (diabetic ketoacidosis)

When you don't get enough insulin over a period of time, your muscle cells become so starved for energy that your body takes emergency measures and breaks down fat. As your body transforms the fat into energy, it produces blood acids known as ketones. A buildup of ketones in the blood is called ketoacidosis (kee-toe-as-ih-DOE-sis).

Diabetic ketoacidosis (DKA) is a dangerous condition that can be fatal if untreated. DKA is more common in people with type 1 diabetes. It can be caused by skipping some of your insulin shots or not raising your dose to adjust for a rise in your blood glucose level.

Extreme stress or illness also may cause DKA to occur in people with either type 1 or type 2 diabetes. When you develop an infection, your body produces

> **?** If I experience diabetic coma and no one is around to help me, will I eventually come out of it?
>
> A comatose condition can result from dangerously high or low blood glucose. Whether consciousness is regained without assistance depends on many factors, including how high or low your blood glucose level is and how long it has been since you last ate or last received an insulin injection. If you live alone or are by yourself for much of the day, recruit family members or friends to give you a call if you don't show up for work or to check on you periodically. It may seem like imposing, but these people are often happy to help, and they may even save your life.

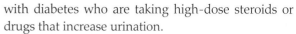

certain hormones, such as adrenaline, to help fight off the problem. Unfortunately, these hormones also work against insulin. Sometimes the extreme stress and illness occur together — you get sick and over-stressed, and you forget to take your insulin.

In people who are unaware they have diabetes, DKA can be the first sign of the disease. Early symptoms of DKA can be confused with the flu, which may delay appropriate medical attention.

What are the signs and symptoms?
As the level of ketones in your blood rises, you may experience:

- High blood glucose
- Excessive thirst
- Dry mouth
- Frequent urination

Later signs and symptoms include:

- Fatigue
- Blurry vision
- Nausea
- Confusion
- Vomiting
- Loss of appetite
- Abdominal pain
- Weight loss
- Shallow breathing
- Weakness
- Sweet, fruity odor on your breath
- Drowsiness

What should you do?
Check your ketone level if you experience any of the signs or symptoms above or whenever your blood glucose is persistently over 250 mg/dL. It's a good idea to also check your ketone level if you're feeling sick or especially stressed.

You can buy a ketones test kit at a drugstore or pharmacy and do the test at home. Most kits use chemically treated strips that you dip into your urine. When you have high amounts of ketones in your blood, excess ketones are excreted in your urine.

Test strips in the kit change color according to the level of ketones in your urine: low, moderate or high. If the color on your test strip shows a moderate or a high ketone level, call your doctor right away for advice on how much insulin to take, and drink plenty of water to prevent dehydration. If you have a high ketone level and you can't reach your doctor, go to the emergency department.

DKA requires emergency medical treatment, which involves replenishing lost fluids through intravenous

(IV) lines. Insulin, which may be combined with glucose, is injected into an IV line so that your body will stop making ketones. Gradually, your blood glucose level is brought back to normal.

Adjusting your blood glucose too quickly can produce swelling in your brain. But this complication appears to be more common in children, especially those with newly diagnosed diabetes.

Left untreated, DKA can lead to a coma and possibly death.

Handling medical emergencies

If your blood sugar goes to extremes (too high or too low), you can have serious problems. Learn the signs below and what to do if they occur. If you have a medical emergency, take action immediately.

Low blood sugar (hypoglycemia)

Early signs and symptoms:
- Sweating
- Shakiness
- Visual disturbances
- Nervousness
- Headache
- Weakness
- Hunger
- Dizziness
- Irritability
- Nausea
- Cold, clammy skin

Later signs and symptoms:
- Slurred speech
- Drowsiness
- Drunken-like behavior
- Confusion

Emergency signs:
- Seizures
- Coma, which can be fatal

What to do:
If blood sugar is below 70 mg/dL, eat or drink something to raise your level quickly, such as hard candy (equal to 5 Life Savers), ½ cup regular (not diet) soft drink, ½ cup fruit juice, or 3 or 4 glucose tablets. If needed, repeat in 15 minutes. If there's no improvement, get medical help right away. If you use insulin, ask your doctor if you should have a glucagon emergency kit.

Dangerously high blood sugar

Early signs and symptoms:
- Excessive thirst
- Leg cramps
- Dry mouth
- Frequent urination
- Dehydration

Later signs and symptoms:
- Rapid pulse
- Weakness
- Confusion

Emergency signs:
- Seizures
- Coma

What to do:
If blood sugar is above 350 mg/dL and you feel ill or stressed, call your doctor for advice. If it's 500 mg/dL or higher, see your doctor immediately.

If your doctor is unable to see you, go to the emergency department. Emergency treatment may correct the problem within hours. Without prompt treatment, the condition can be fatal.

Older adults with diabetes who don't get enough fluids are at particular risk.

High ketones (diabetic ketoacidosis)

Early signs and symptoms:
- High blood sugar
- Dry mouth
- Excessive thirst
- Frequent urination

Later signs and symptoms:
- Fatigue
- Nausea
- Vomiting
- Abdominal pain
- Shallow breathing
- Sweet, fruity odor on your breath
- Blurry vision
- Confusion
- Loss of appetite
- Weight loss
- Weakness
- Drowsiness

Emergency signs:
- Seizures
- Coma

What to do:
Check your ketone level, especially if blood sugar is persistently above 250 mg/dL. If the test strip color shows a moderate or high ketone level, call your doctor right away and ask how much insulin to take. Drink plenty of water to prevent dehydration. If your ketone level is high and you can't reach your doctor, go to the emergency department.

Long-term complications

Long-term diabetes complications develop gradually and may lead to other disabling or life-threatening diseases.

Heart and blood vessel disease

Heart and blood vessel disease (cardiovascular disease) is the leading cause of death among people with diabetes. Diabetes can damage your major arteries as well as your small blood vessels, making it easier for fatty deposits (plaques) to form in arteries, a condition called atherosclerosis (ath-ur-o-skluh-ROE-sis). This narrowing of the arteries causes an increased risk of a heart attack, stroke and other disorders from impaired circulation.

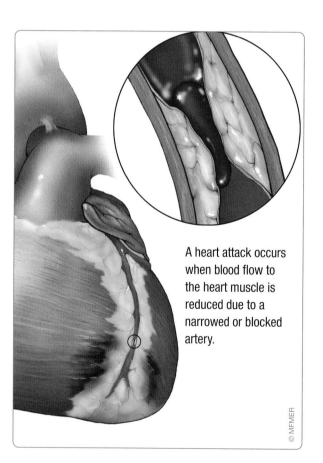

A heart attack occurs when blood flow to the heart muscle is reduced due to a narrowed or blocked artery.

© MFMER

Silent heart attacks

If you have diabetes, you're at particular risk of silent (asymptomatic) heart attacks — heart attacks without typical symptoms. Diabetes can damage nerves that transmit chest pain, which typically accompanies a heart attack.

Without pain sensations, you may be unaware that a heart attack is occurring. Even without diabetes, many women and older adults often don't have the classic early warning signs of a heart attack, such as chest pain. Still, the more signs and symptoms you have, the more likely you're having a heart attack.

Coronary artery disease

Coronary artery disease is caused by atherosclerosis in blood vessels that feed your heart (coronary arteries). Over time, fatty deposits can narrow your coronary arteries, so less oxygen-rich blood flows to your heart muscle. Once a blockage is severe enough, heart muscle can be damaged due to a lack of oxygen (ischemia), causing a heart attack.

Signs and symptoms

Signs and symptoms of coronary artery disease vary, as does severity, depending on the extent of the disease and the individual. In its early stages, coronary artery disease often produces no symptoms. Later on, you may experience signs and symptoms such as:

▶ Shortness of breath
▶ Fatigue
▶ Rapid or irregular heartbeats (palpitations)

Or you may have warning signs of a heart attack.

Heart attack

You could be having a heart attack if you have any of these signs or symptoms:

▶ Pressure, fullness or squeezing pain in the center of your chest for more than a few minutes
▶ Pain extending beyond your chest to your shoulder, arm, back, or your teeth and jaw

- Increasing or prolonged episodes of chest pain
- Prolonged pain in the upper abdomen
- Shortness of breath
- Sweating
- Impending sense of doom
- Lightheadedness
- Fainting
- Nausea and vomiting

If you think you're having a heart attack, immediately call 911 or a local emergency number. Damage to your heart from a heart attack increases your risk of developing heart failure.

Stroke

A stroke occurs when the blood supply to a part of your brain is interrupted or severely reduced and brain tissue is deprived of essential oxygen and nutrients. Within a few minutes to a few hours, brain cells begin to die.

The interruption can be from a clogged or blocked artery (ischemic stroke) or from a leaking or ruptured artery (hemorrhagic stroke). Ischemic stroke is much more common.

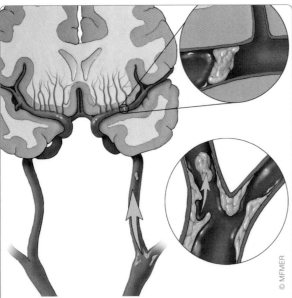

A stroke most often results when a brain artery becomes clogged or blocked by fatty deposits (plaques), reducing blood flow.

Signs and symptoms

The most common signs and symptoms include:

- Sudden numbness, weakness or paralysis of the face, arm or leg — usually on one side of the body
- Loss of speech, or trouble talking or understanding speech
- Sudden blurred, double or decreased vision
- Dizziness, loss of balance or loss of coordination
- A sudden, severe or unusual headache, possibly with a stiff neck, facial pain, pain between the eyes, vomiting or altered consciousness
- Confusion, or problems with memory, spatial orientation or perception.

If you think you're having a stroke, immediately call 911 or a local emergency number.

Nerve damage (neuropathy)

Nerve damage, also called neuropathy (noo-ROP-uh-thee), is a common long-term complication of diabetes. Within your body is a complex network of nerves, connecting your brain to muscles, skin and other organs. Through these nerves, your brain senses pain, controls your muscles, and performs automatic tasks such as breathing and digestion.

High blood glucose levels can damage delicate nerves. Excess glucose is thought to weaken the walls of tiny blood vessels (capillaries) that nourish your nerves. Diabetic neuropathy affects about half of all people with diabetes. Sometimes the results can be painful and disabling. More often the symptoms are mild.

Signs and symptoms

There are many kinds of nerve damage:

- Damage to your sensory nerves may leave you unable to detect sensations such as pain, warmth, coolness and texture.
- Damage to your autonomic nerves can increase your heart rate and perspiration level. In men, such damage can interfere with their ability to have an erection.
- Damage to nerves that control your muscles may leave you with weakened muscles and loss of strength.

Most commonly, diabetes damages the sensory nerves in your legs, and less often, your arms. You may

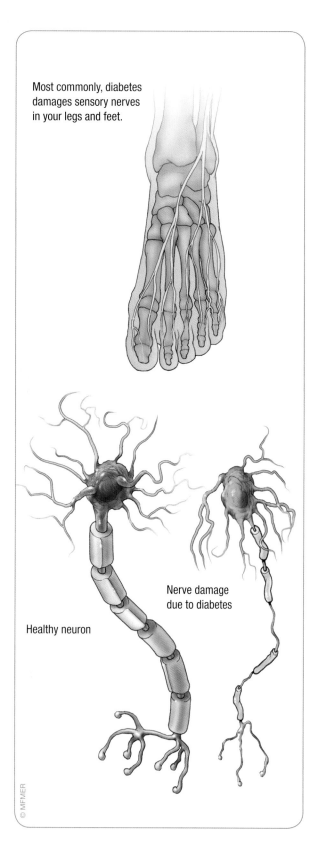

Most commonly, diabetes damages sensory nerves in your legs and feet.

Healthy neuron

Nerve damage due to diabetes

© MFMER

experience any of these symptoms, which often begin at the tips of your toes, fingers or both and gradually spread upward:

▶ A tingling feeling, numbness, pain or a combination of these sensations
▶ Burning pain that comes and goes
▶ Stabbing or aching pain that's worse at night
▶ A crawling sensation

Left untreated, symptoms of decreased sensation can progress, putting you at high risk of injuring your feet without realizing it. Minor injuries, when not recognized early, can lead to bigger problems.

Kidney disease (nephropathy)

Each of your kidneys has about a million nephrons. A nephron is a tiny filtering unit with tiny blood vessels (capillaries) that remove waste from your blood and send it to your urine.

Diabetes can damage this delicate filtering system, often before you notice any symptoms. Up to 40 percent of people with diabetes eventually develop kidney disease, called nephropathy (nuh-FROP-uh-thee). The longer you have diabetes, the higher your risk of eventually experiencing damage to your kidneys.

Signs and symptoms

In its early stages, kidney disease produces few symptoms. Generally, damage is extensive before these signs and symptoms occur:

▶ Swelling of the ankles, feet and hands
▶ Shortness of breath
▶ High blood pressure
▶ Confusion or difficulty concentrating
▶ Poor appetite
▶ Metallic taste in your mouth
▶ Fatigue

Eye damage (retinopathy)

Many tiny vessels nourish the back part of your eye, called the retina. These blood vessels are often among the first to be damaged by high blood glucose. This damage is called diabetic retinopathy (ret-ih-NOP-uh-thee).

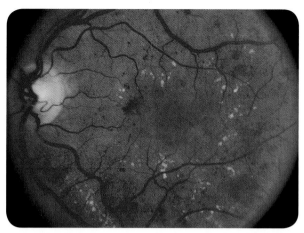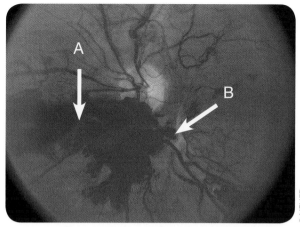

In nonproliferative diabetic retinopathy (left), engorged blood vessels, tiny red dots (microaneurysms), large red dots (hemorrhages) and yellow spots (exudates) are common. In advanced-stage proliferative diabetic retinopathy (right), abnormal blood vessels can grow on the optic nerve and retina. These blood vessels can break, causing massive hemorrhages (A) and the formation of scar tissue (B).

Nearly everyone with type 1 diabetes and more than 6 out of 10 people with type 2 diabetes develop some form of eye damage by the time they've had diabetes for 20 years. Most people experience only mild problems. For others, the effects are more severe.

Types

There are two types of diabetic retinopathy.

Nonproliferative This form is mild and more common. Blood vessels in your retina become weak and may swell or develop bulges or fatty deposits. The condition generally doesn't affect your vision unless swollen vessels form in the tiny portion of your retina called the macula.

Proliferative When tiny blood vessels in the retina are damaged, they can bleed or close off. New and fragile blood vessels may form (proliferate) in the retina, and they too may bleed. If the bleeding is heavy or occurs in certain areas of the eye, it can damage your retina and distort your vision, possibly leading to blindness.

Signs and symptoms

Early diabetic retinopathy often produces few, if any, visual symptoms. As the damage becomes more severe, these symptoms may develop:

- "Spiders," "cobwebs" or tiny specks floating in your vision
- Blurred vision
- A dark or empty spot in the center of your vision
- Dark streaks or a red film that blocks vision
- Flashes of light
- Poor night vision
- Vision loss
- Increased risk of infection

High blood glucose impairs the ability of your immune cells to fight off invading germs and bacteria, putting you at higher risk of infection. Your mouth, gums, lungs, skin, feet, bladder and genital area are common infection sites.

Signs and symptoms of infection vary, depending on its location. A low-grade fever is common with many infections.

Chapter 2
Monitoring Your Blood Sugar

How often and when to test 32

What you'll need 33

Performing the test 35

Advances in monitoring tools 36

Recording your results 38

Keeping within your range 40

Troubleshooting problems 41

Factors that affect blood glucose levels 43

When test results signal a problem 46

Avoiding the highs and lows 46

Overcoming barriers 49

A visit with Nancy Klobassa-Davidson

"The primary reason that people respond to monitoring in the manner they do is fear. And this fear is usually related to a lack of accurate information about blood sugar testing."

"My doctor just told me that I have diabetes, and if that isn't bad enough, now I find out that I have to test my blood sugar. That means I have to prick my finger with a needle, doesn't it? I've had that done before, and it hurts. Isn't there some other way to test my blood sugar? Besides, my diabetes isn't that bad. And I feel fine. Now, if I was on insulin, then my diabetes would be more serious. Then I would have to test my blood sugar, right?"

As a diabetes educator, I frequently hear many of these comments when someone who's just been diagnosed with diabetes finds out that he or she needs to begin blood sugar (glucose) monitoring. The primary reason people respond to monitoring in the manner that they do is fear. And this fear is usually related to a lack of accurate information about blood sugar testing. Certainly, it's normal to be afraid of something new — particularly for a procedure that may cause some discomfort — such as monitoring your blood sugar. However, most people find the procedure isn't nearly as difficult and painful as they imagined, and after a while it simply becomes routine.

A useful approach I use when working with an individual who is fearful about testing his or her blood sugar is to do the test at the beginning of the education session. The person finds out that the procedure causes only mild discomfort, and testing right away means he or she won't have to sit through the session anticipating the finger stick. I explain that the needles (lancets) are very fine and are coated with silicone, which reduces the discomfort associated with a finger stick. Then we talk about how there are fewer nerve endings on the sides of the finger than on the fingertip pads. I also tell the person there is no other way to obtain a blood sample without using a needle on some area of the body.

People with newly diagnosed diabetes often want to know why it's so important to monitor their blood

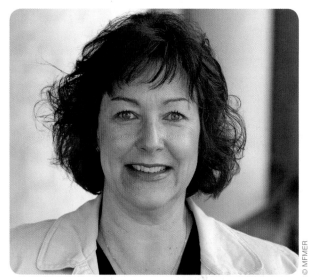

Nancy M. Klobassa-Davidson
Diabetes Educator, Endocrinology

sugar. The answer is that monitoring provides valuable information in regard to how exercise, food, medications, stress and many other factors affect blood sugar.

Finally, I like to remind my patients that blood glucose monitoring is just a tool. Your blood sugar is only a number and not a reflection of you as a person. If you have days when your blood sugar doesn't fall within your desirable range, it doesn't mean that you've failed. Everyone has bad days now and then. The goal is for you to do the best you can so that you can enjoy good health.

Control. That word comes up again and again, and for good reason. If you have diabetes, controlling your blood sugar (glucose) level is the single most important thing you can do to feel your best and prevent long-term complications.

But how do you achieve control? The cornerstones to controlling diabetes include five basic steps:

▶ Monitoring your blood glucose
▶ Eating a varied and healthy diet
▶ Staying active
▶ Maintaining a healthy weight
▶ Using medications appropriately, when necessary

This chapter focuses on the first of these five behaviors. Blood glucose monitoring is essential — it's the only way to know whether you're achieving your treatment goals.

If you've just been diagnosed with diabetes, or your treatment has changed, monitoring can seem overwhelming at first. You might feel angry, upset or fearful about having diabetes. You may be anxious about testing — afraid that it will take over your life, that it will be painful or disruptive. These feelings are normal.

But as you learn how to measure your blood glucose and understand how regular testing can help you, you'll feel more comfortable with the procedure and more in control of your disease.

Your doctor or a diabetes educator can help you determine a monitoring schedule that's right for you.

How often and when to test

How often you need to test your blood glucose and at what time of day depend on the type of diabetes you have and your treatment plan. If you take insulin, you should test your blood glucose frequently, at least twice a day. Your doctor may advise testing three or four times a day or even more often.

Testing is commonly done before meals and at bedtime — in other words, when you haven't eaten for four or more hours. Your doctor may also advise you to check your blood glucose level one to two hours after a meal. It's generally best to test your blood glucose just before your insulin injection.

A change in your regular routine may be another reason to test your blood glucose, especially if you have type 1 diabetes. This may include exercising more than normal, eating less than usual or traveling. Special circumstances, including pregnancy or illness, also may warrant increased testing.

If you have type 2 diabetes and you don't need insulin, test your blood glucose as often as necessary to make sure it's under control. For some people this may mean daily testing, while for others it might be twice a week.

In general, if you're able to control your blood glucose with diet and exercise and without using medication, you probably won't need to test your blood sugar as often. However, it's still important that you keep track of your blood sugar levels.

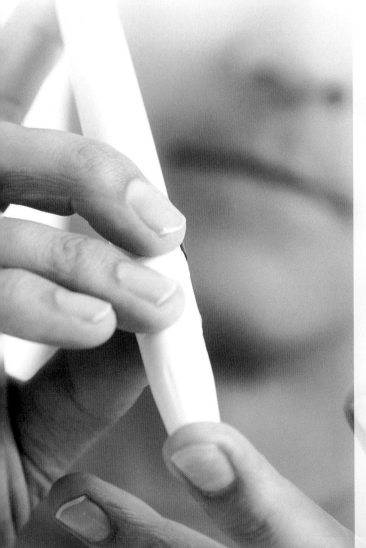

What you'll need

1. Lancet
2. Cap for finger sticks
3. Cap for alternate site sticks
4. Blood glucose meter
5. Lancing device
6. Test strip vial
7. Test strip

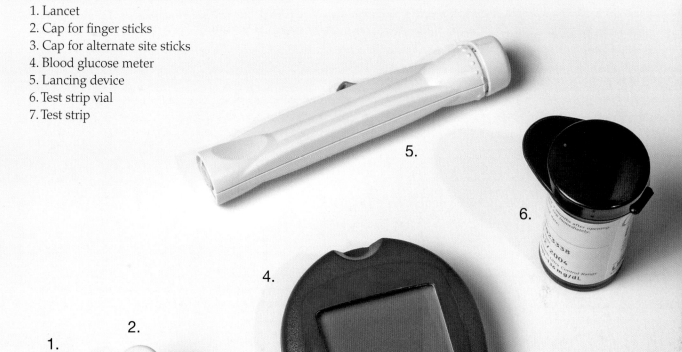

Testing your blood glucose is a quick and easy process that generally takes less than two minutes. Some tools you'll need include:

Lancet and lancing device

A lancet is a small needle that pricks the skin on your finger so that you can draw a drop of blood. A lancing device holds the lancet. Spring-loaded lancing devices are generally less painful than are other types. Because people differ in skin thickness, lancets can usually be set for different prick depths.

Test strips

Test strips are chemically treated — you place blood from your finger (or another site) on these strips. You'll insert the strip into the device first, before drawing blood.

Blood glucose meter

A blood glucose meter, also called a blood glucose monitor, is a small, computerized device that measures and displays your blood glucose level. These meters come in many forms (see page 34).

Choosing the right meter

Blood glucose meters come in many forms with a variety of features. So how do you know which device is right for you? Your diabetes educator or doctor may recommend a meter or help you select one. Keep in mind that some health plans require their participants to use a specific meter. When choosing a meter, consider these factors:

Cost

Most insurance plans and Medicare cover the cost of a blood glucose meter and test strips (after you pay your deductible and any coinsurance). Find out what your insurance covers before you buy. Some plans limit the total number of test strips allowed. Meters vary widely in price, so shop around before you buy. The test strips are the most expensive part of monitoring because they're used so often. Figure out which type of strip is most cost-effective for you.

Ease of use and maintenance

Some meters are easier to use than are others. Are the meter and strips comfortable to hold? Can you easily see the numbers on the screen? How easy is it to get blood onto the strips? Does it require a small or large drop of blood? Most meters use cell batteries, which last a long time. A battery symbol shows up on the screen when the battery is low and needs to be changed.

Special features

Ask about the features to see what meets your specific needs. For example, some meters are large with strips that are easier to handle. Some are compact and easier to carry. Others have a backlight or audio capability. People with impaired vision can buy a meter with a large screen or a "talking" meter that announces the results. For children there are colorful meters that give a quick reading.

Some meters include rechargeable batteries that work with a wall or computer charger. Recharging is generally needed every one to two weeks.

Also consider how the meter stores and retrieves information. Many track the time and date of a test, the result, and trends over time. One type of meter tracks high and low blood glucose patterns within preset target ranges. You can download this information into a computer to chart your diabetes management.

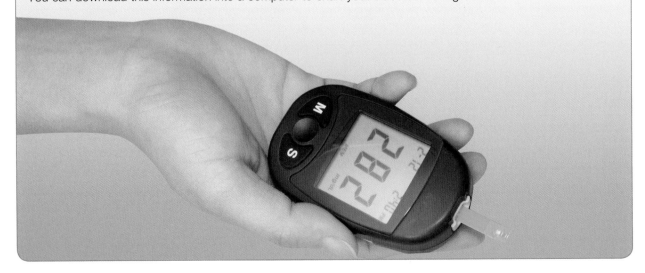

Performing the test

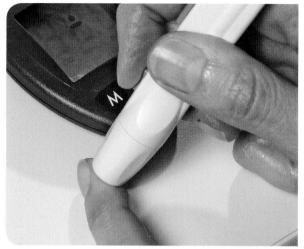

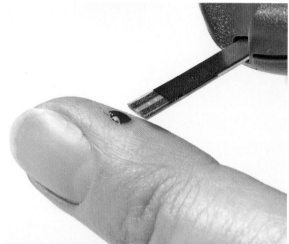

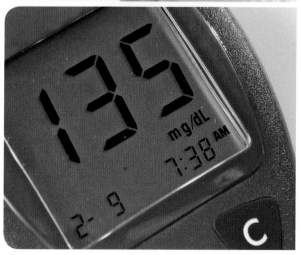

Once you have the right equipment, you're ready to start testing your blood glucose on the schedule recommended by your doctor.

Testing basics

It's important to follow the instructions that come with your particular glucose meter. In general, here's how the process works:

- Before pricking your finger, wash your hands with soap and warm water. Then dry them well.
- Remove a test strip from the container and replace the cap immediately to prevent damage to the strips.
- Insert the test strip into the meter.
- Place the tip of the lancet on your finger. Stick the side of your finger, not the tip, so that you won't have sore spots on the part of your finger you use the most.
- Hold your hand down to encourage a drop of blood to form. When you have a drop of blood, carefully touch the test strip to the blood (but avoid touching your skin with the test strip) and wait for a reading.
- Within a few seconds, the meter will display your blood glucose level on a screen.

Other recommendations from experts

Your fingertips contain a lot of nerve endings, so make sure to rotate the sites where you stick your fingers to minimize any discomfort.

If you have a newer glucose meter, you'll have the option to test your blood glucose from other sites, such as your forearm, palm or thigh. But check with your doctor or diabetes educator first to find out if alternate site testing is appropriate in your case. Read more about alternate site testing on pages 36 and 37.

Advances in monitoring tools

Although finger pricks remain the gold standard for blood sugar monitoring, researchers are developing products designed to take the "ouch" out of the process. You might ask your diabetes educator about these potential alternatives and if they would be an option for you.

Device	How it works	Considerations
Alternate site monitor	Most blood glucose meters are approved for alternate site testing. An alternate site monitor allows you to take blood samples from areas likely to be less painful than your finger, such as your arm, palm or thigh.	Blood samples from alternate sites are not as accurate as fingertip samples when your blood sugar level is rising or falling quickly.
Continuous glucose monitor	A continuous glucose monitor (CGM) uses a sensor to measure blood sugar levels in fluid under the skin. CGM readings are transmitted to a small recording device worn on your body or to a compatible insulin pump. An alarm can warn you if your blood sugar level becomes too low or too high. Blood sugar readings and trends can be downloaded to a computer and viewed by you and your health care providers.	Sensors cost between $35 and $100 each and must be changed every three to seven days. CGM readings can supplement blood glucose meter information — you'll still need to check your blood sugar levels two to four times a day with a traditional monitor.
Disposable glucose meter	Disposable meters have test strips built into the vial cap. They can be a good option if you forget or lose your regular meter or to use while traveling.	The cost of a disposable meter is about the same as a vial of test strips.

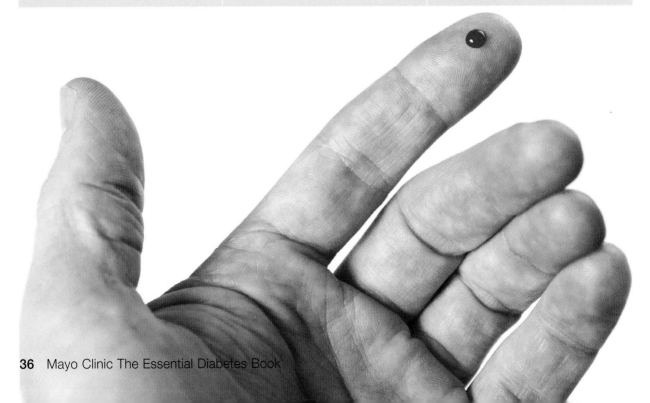

Alternate site testing

Newer glucose meters offer what's called alternate site testing. That means you can test your blood from sites other than the fingertip — such as the palm, forearm, upper arm and thigh. But the Food and Drug Administration (FDA) points out that blood from your fingertips shows changes in blood glucose levels (after a meal or exercise, for example) more quickly than does blood from other sites. In other words, results from other sites may not always be as accurate.

Use blood from your finger rather than other sites if:

▶ You think your blood glucose is low
▶ Your blood glucose is rapidly changing because of food or medication
▶ You've just finished exercising
▶ You suspect that the results from the alternative site are unreliable

When using an alternate site, you'll need to massage the puncture site to stimulate the flow of blood before you use the lancing device. Check the instructions that come with the glucose meter to see which sites the FDA approved for the product you're using. Ask your doctor or diabetes educator if it's acceptable to use sites other than your fingertip.

? What's the difference between whole blood glucose levels and plasma glucose levels?

Home glucose meters use whole blood to measure glucose levels. But when blood is drawn at your medical appointment and sent to a lab, the red blood cells are removed, leaving only plasma, before glucose is measured.

Because of this difference, results from labs and home monitors aren't exactly the same. Plasma tests tend to be more accurate, and the results are 10 to 15 percent higher than are whole blood test results. But most home meters (especially new ones) are calibrated to give a plasma test result, even though they use whole blood for the test. Your home monitor's results are considered accurate if they fall within 15 percent of the lab test result.

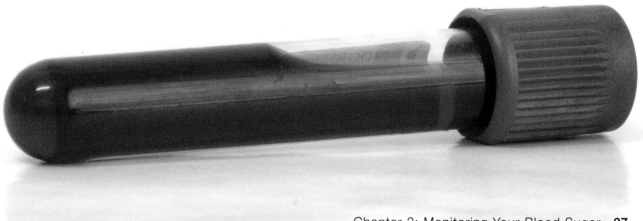

Recording your results

More than just providing an immediate measurement of your blood glucose, blood sugar monitoring can help you assess your progress in managing your diabetes.

Each time you perform a blood test, log your results. This information helps you see how food, physical activity, medication and other factors affect your blood glucose. As patterns occur, you can begin to understand how your daily activities affect your blood sugar levels. This puts you in a better position to manage your diabetes day by day and even hour by hour.

Your life is not the same from one day to the next. Some days you exercise more or eat less. Maybe you're sick or you're having trouble at work or at

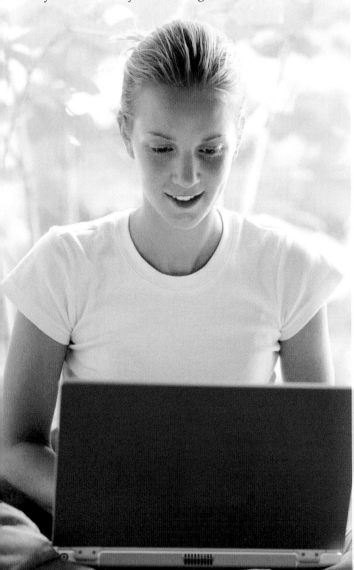

home. Changes such as these can affect your blood glucose level.

By keeping an accurate record of both day-to-day events and your blood glucose levels, you may identify some problem areas for you. By addressing these areas you'll be better able to maintain good blood glucose control.

With the information you gain, you can even learn how to anticipate problems before they occur. You can plan ahead for changes in your routine that you know will affect your blood glucose levels. This may include activities such as traveling, eating out or exercising harder than usual.

What to track

A diabetes educator or your doctor may have given you a record book for recording your test results. If not, you can use any type of notebook. You can also keep your results on a computer. Many software programs are available for recording and tracking blood glucose levels — ask your health care team what they recommend.

Every time you check your blood glucose, record:

▶ The date and time
▶ The test result
▶ The type and dosage of medication you're taking

Also include information that can help explain a change from your normal blood glucose level, such as:

▶ A change in your diet (for example, having a birthday dinner, eating at a restaurant or eating more than usual)
▶ A change in your exercise or activity level
▶ Unusual excitement or stress
▶ An illness
▶ An insulin reaction

Take your records and blood glucose meter with you when you see your doctor, diabetes educator or dietitian. He or she can help you interpret the results. Based on the information that you track, your doctor may recommend changes in your medication and discuss your diet, level of physical activity and other lifestyle issues. The more complete your records are, the more useful they'll be.

Date	Medication dose	Blood glucose test results				Comments*
		Before break-fast meal	Before noon meal	Before eve-ning meal	Bedtime	

*Changes in diet and activity, weight, insulin reactions, illness, urine ketones, and so on

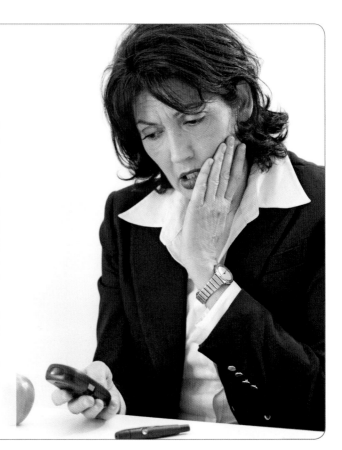
Keeping within your range

As you check and record your blood glucose levels, you want your blood sugar to stay within a desirable range — not too high or too low. This range is often referred to as your target range or your blood glucose goal.

The normal range for a fasting blood glucose level is 70 to 100 milligrams of glucose per deciliter of blood (mg/dL). Ideally, that's the level at which you want to keep your blood glucose before meals. But that's not realistic for most people with diabetes. Instead, your focus may be on a range that's near normal. Your doctor will help you determine your blood glucose goals.

Because blood glucose naturally rises after eating, your goal after meals will be different from that before meals. Your goal before bed also may be different from during the day.

In determining what blood glucose goals to recommend for you, your doctor takes into account several factors, including your age, whether you have any diabetes-related complications or other medical conditions, and how good you are at recognizing when your blood glucose is low.

Recognizing the signs and symptoms of low blood glucose (hypoglycemia) is important because if your blood glucose drops too low, you may lose consciousness or have a seizure. See page 48 for more information on the warning signs of hypoglycemia.

These are the blood sugar goals adults with diabetes generally aim to meet:

- Before meals — 90 to 130 mg/dL
- About 1 to 2 hours after a meal — Under 180 mg/dL
- Before bedtime — 110 to 150 mg/dL

Your goals may differ, especially if you have complications, you're pregnant or you're older — so always follow the advice of your doctor.

Troubleshooting problems

Blood glucose meters are generally accurate and precise. Human error rather than a nonfunctioning machine is more likely to produce an inaccurate meter reading.

If you think something's not right with your readings, start with the basics.

Check the test strips

Throw out damaged or outdated strips.

Check the meter

Make sure the meter is at room temperature, and the strip guide and the test window are clean. Replace the batteries in the meter, if needed.

To check your meter and your testing skill, take the device along when you visit your doctor or have an appointment for lab work. Your doctor or diabetes educator can have you check your blood glucose at the same time that blood is drawn for lab tests. That way, you can compare the reading you get with the lab results.

Check the measurement scale (calibration)

Some meters must be calibrated to each container of test strips. Be sure the code number in the device matches the code number on the container of test strips.

Your meter results shouldn't be off by more than 15 percent. In addition, once a week, do a quality control test of your equipment and technique. It's also a good idea to do the test when you start a new container of test strips or you calibrate the meter or change the batteries.

To do a quality control test, follow your normal blood-testing procedure, but use a liquid control solution instead of blood. These solutions are available at most drugstores and pharmacies and come in three ranges: high, normal or low. Ask your diabetes educator which solution to use.

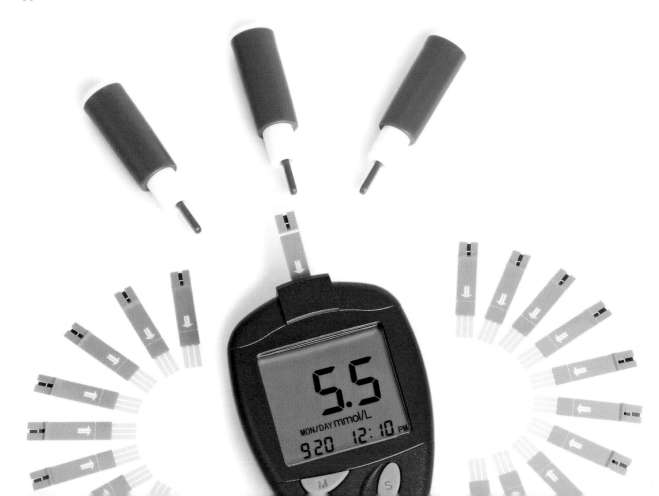

Check your technique

Wash your hands with soap and water before pricking your finger. Apply a generous drop of blood to the test strip. Don't add more blood to the test strip after the first drop was applied.

Check for other problems

Other problems that can lead to an inaccurate reading include:

▶ Not enough blood applied to the test strip
▶ More blood added to the test strip after the first drop was applied
▶ Alcohol, dirt or other substances on your finger or alternative site
▶ A meter that's not at room temperature
▶ A damaged meter

After you've corrected potential problems, repeat the control test. If the results are still unacceptable, talk to your diabetes educator or call the meter manufacturer for help.

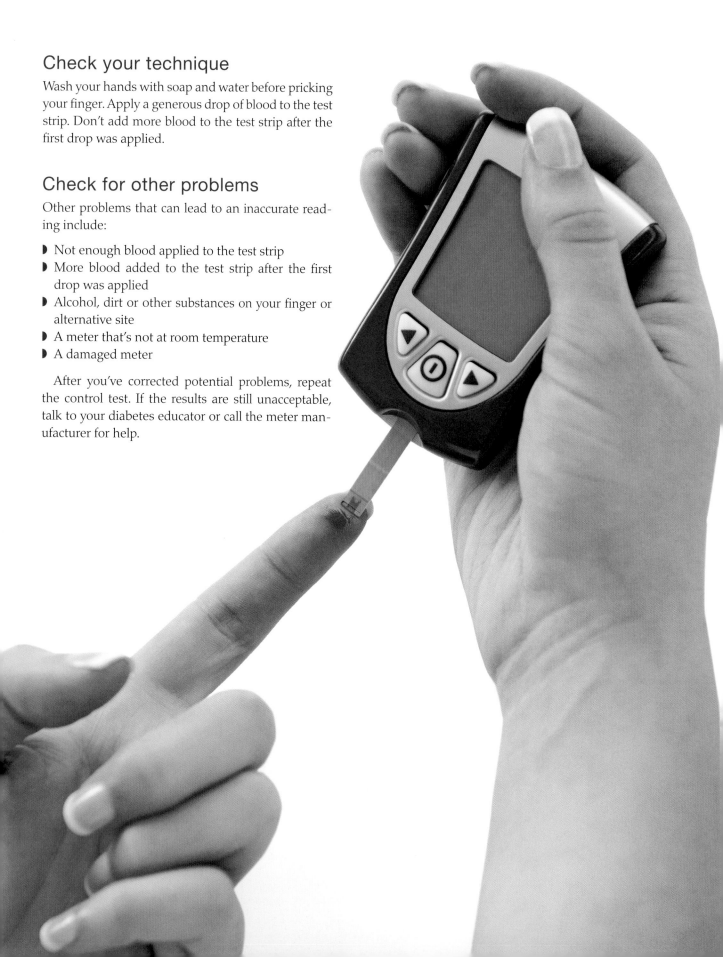

Factors that affect blood glucose levels

The amount of glucose in your blood continuously varies. That's because many factors affect how your body metabolizes food into glucose and how it uses this glucose. Self-monitoring helps you learn what makes your blood sugar level rise and fall so that you can make adjustments in your treatment. It can also help you understand why your blood glucose level may be different from day to day or hour to hour.

Food

The food you eat raises your blood glucose level. One to two hours after a meal, your blood glucose is at its highest level. Then it starts to fall. What you eat, how much you eat and at what time of day you eat all affect your blood glucose level. Strive for consistency from day to day in the time you eat and the amount of food you eat.

By controlling when and how much you eat, you control the times your blood glucose is higher, such as after meals. You also control how high your blood glucose rises.

If you eat too much, your blood glucose will be higher than usual. Too little food may result in lower than usual blood sugar. If you take insulin, this could put you at risk of hypoglycemia. It's also important to understand that different foods have different effects on your blood glucose.

Food is made up of carbohydrates, protein and fat. All increase blood glucose, but carbohydrates have the most noticeable effect. Within the carbohydrates group, different types have varying effects.

Your liver

As mentioned in Chapter 1, glucose is stored in your liver in the form of glycogen. Your liver also makes new glucose from other substances, such as protein and fat.

When your blood glucose level falls, your liver breaks down glycogen and releases it into your bloodstream. This generally happens when you haven't eaten for a while. The process of storing and releasing glucose causes natural variations in blood glucose levels, but it's more pronounced when you have diabetes.

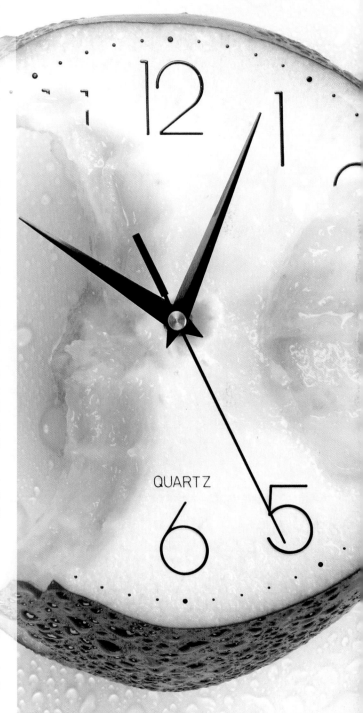

Exercise and physical activity

Typically, exercise and physical activity lower your blood glucose level. With help from insulin, exercise

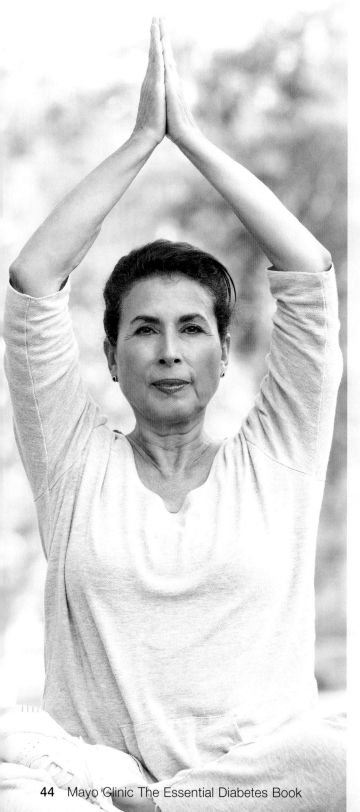

and physical activity promote the transfer of glucose from your blood to your cells, where the glucose is used for energy. The more you exercise, the more glucose you use and the faster it's transported to cells, lowering the amount of glucose in your blood. Exercise also makes your cells more responsive to insulin, so it works more efficiently.

Although fairly uncommon, sometimes exercise has the opposite effect — it raises your blood glucose. This usually happens if your blood glucose is very high to begin with.

Until you know how your body responds to exercise, test your blood glucose before and after exercising and again several hours later.

Medications

Insulin and oral diabetes medications lower your blood glucose level. The time of day you take your medication and how much you take affect how much your blood glucose level drops. If your medication is causing your blood glucose to drop too much, or not enough, your doctor may need to make adjustments to your dosage.

Medications taken for other conditions also can affect blood glucose. Whenever you're prescribed a new medication for another health condition, remind your doctor that you have diabetes and ask if the medication may alter your blood glucose level.

By being aware of a medication's effects and following simple precautions, such as increased glucose monitoring, you may keep it from causing significant changes in your blood glucose levels. If the drug does make it harder for you to control your blood glucose, talk with your doctor.

Illness

The physical stress of a cold, the flu or another illness, especially a bacterial infection, causes your body to produce hormones that increase blood glucose. Injury or a serious health problem such as a heart attack also can increase your blood glucose level.

The additional glucose helps to promote healing. But in people with diabetes, more glucose can be a problem. When you're sick it's important to monitor your blood glucose frequently.

Alcohol

Alcohol prevents your liver from releasing glucose and can increase the risk of your blood glucose falling too low. If you take insulin or oral diabetes medications and you drink alcohol, you risk experiencing low blood glucose (hypoglycemia). This is true even with as little as 2 ounces. If you choose to drink alcohol, drink only in moderation.

To prevent your blood glucose from dropping too low, never drink on an empty stomach or if your blood glucose is already low. (See "Diabetes and alcohol: Do they mix?" on page 66.)

Less commonly, alcohol can do the opposite — cause your blood glucose to rise. This could happen, for example, with the sugary sodas or juices used in mixed drinks. Monitor your blood glucose before and after drinking alcohol to see how your body responds to its use.

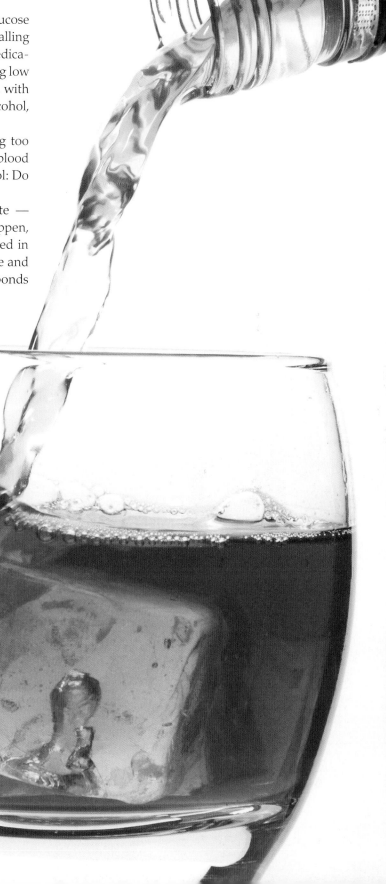

What about stress?

Stress can affect blood glucose in two ways. When you're under a lot of stress, it's easy to abandon your usual routine. You may exercise less, eat less healthy foods and not test your blood sugar as often. As a result, stress indirectly may cause your blood glucose to rise.

Occasionally, stress can have a direct effect on your blood glucose level. Physical and psychological stress may cause your body to produce hormones that prevent insulin from working properly, increasing blood glucose levels. This tends to be more common in people with type 2 diabetes.

To find out how you react to stress, log your stress level on a scale of 1 to 10 every time you log your blood glucose level. After a couple of weeks, look for a pattern. Do high blood glucose levels often occur with high stress levels and low blood glucose levels with low stress? If so, stress may be affecting your blood glucose control — discuss this with your doctor or diabetes educator.

When test results signal a problem

Watch for patterns that show that your blood glucose readings are persistently above or below your goals. This might indicate that your medication needs to be adjusted. If you're not taking medication and your glucose levels are above your goals, it may indicate that your diet and exercise efforts aren't enough and medication is warranted.

Persistently high or low blood glucose readings put you at risk of complications of diabetes, which were discussed in Chapter 1. Experiencing high or low blood glucose levels once in a while — especially if you can identify the reason — isn't cause for alarm. However, frequent, unexplained high or low readings need attention.

It's important to call your doctor if:

▶ Your blood glucose is persistently higher than 300 mg/dL
▶ Your blood glucose readings are persistently above or below your goals
▶ Your blood glucose is greater than 250 mg/dL for more than 24 hours during an illness
▶ You frequently have signs and symptoms of low blood glucose (hypoglycemia)

Avoiding the highs and lows

Blood sugar levels that are out of your target range can cause a problem, especially if the levels are very high or very low. Here's what to watch for and how to react.

High blood sugar

Everyone has occasional episodes of high blood sugar — what's known as hyperglycemia. Still, hyperglycemia is nothing to take lightly.

If you have diabetes, your mouth feels dry and you've been thirsty all day, check your blood sugar. When you do, you may discover it's a lot higher than your target range.

The most common causes of hypoglycemia include:

▶ Eating too much food or the wrong foods
▶ Exercising too little
▶ Physical stress, such as an infection or other illness
▶ Emotional stress, such as family conflict or workplace challenges
▶ Forgetting to take your oral diabetes medication
▶ Problems with your insulin, such as not giving yourself enough insulin or using expired insulin

What to watch for
Paying attention to the early signs and symptoms of hyperglycemia can help you get control of the condition promptly.

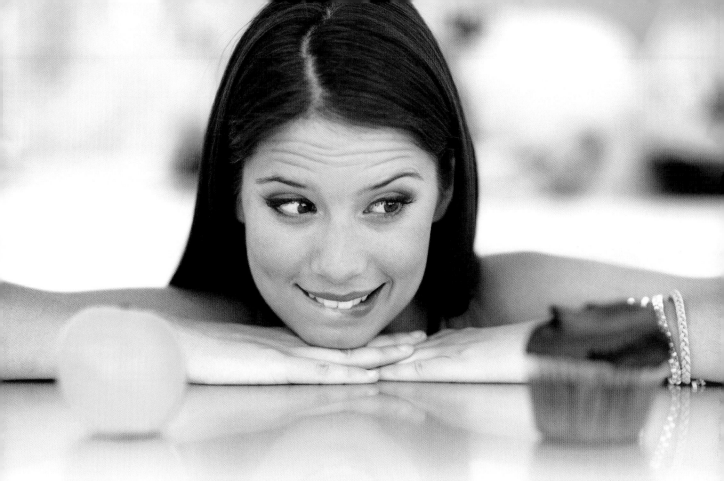

Watch for these common warning signs:

- Frequent urination
- Increased thirst
- Blurred vision
- Fatigue

If your blood sugar level climbs high enough, you may develop diabetic ketoacidosis or hyperglycemic hyperosmolar syndrome. When you have diabetic ketoacidosis, your body begins to break down fat for energy. This produces toxic acids known as ketones.

When you have hyperglycemic hyperosmolar syndrome, your blood becomes thick and syrupy. Left untreated, both conditions are life-threatening.

What to do

If you experience any signs or symptoms of hyperglycemia — even if they're subtle — check your blood sugar level. If your blood sugar level is higher than normal, use a home test kit to check your urine for ketones. If the urine test is positive, your body may have started making the changes that can lead to diabetic ketoacidosis. You'll need your doctor's help to safely lower your blood sugar level.

If there are no ketones in your urine, you may be able to treat hyperglycemia on your own.

- **Take your medication as directed.** If you have frequent episodes of hyperglycemia, your doctor may adjust the dosage or timing of your medication.
- **Get physical.** Exercise is often an effective way to lower blood sugar. But there's a caveat. If you have ketones in your urine, exercise can drive your blood sugar even higher.
- **Eat less.** It helps to eat less and avoid sugary beverages. If you're having trouble sticking to your meal plan, ask your doctor or dietitian for help.

Prevention steps

Long periods of hyperglycemia aren't good. They can damage your nerves, blood vessels and many organs.

You can prevent these complications by following your diabetes treatment plan and by treating episodes of high blood sugar quickly. Work with your diabetes treatment team to make sure your diabetes treatment plan is meeting your needs.

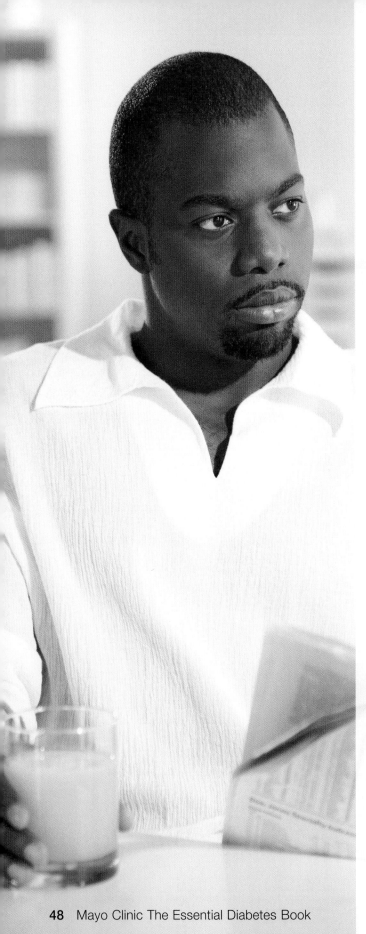

Low blood sugar

Hypoglycemia — often defined as blood sugar below 70 milligrams per deciliter (mg/dL) or 4 millimoles per liter (mmol/L) — occurs when there's too much insulin and not enough sugar (glucose) in your blood. Hypoglycemia is most common among people who take insulin, but it can also occur if you're taking oral diabetes medications. Culprits may include:

◗ Taking too much diabetes medication
◗ Not eating enough
◗ Postponing or skipping a meal
◗ Increasing physical activity without eating more
◗ Drinking alcohol

What to watch for

Paying attention to the early signs and symptoms of hypoglycemia can help you treat the condition promptly. Red flags include:

◗ Shakiness
◗ Clumsiness
◗ Dizziness
◗ Weakness
◗ Sweating
◗ Hunger

◗ Irritability or moodiness
◗ Headache
◗ Blurry or double vision
◗ Pounding heartbeat
◗ Confusion

If you develop hypoglycemia during the night, you might wake to sweat-soaked pajamas or a headache.

It's important to take your warning signs seriously. Hypoglycemia can increase the risk of serious — even deadly — accidents. Left untreated, hypoglycemia can lead to seizures and loss of consciousness. Rarely, severe hypoglycemia can be fatal.

What to do

If you think that your blood sugar may be dipping too low, check your blood sugar level. If the results confirm that you're experiencing hypoglycemia, then eat or drink something that will raise your blood sugar level quickly. This includes:

◗ Five to six pieces of hard candy
◗ Four ounces fruit juice
◗ Five to 6 ounces regular — not diet — soda
◗ One tablespoon sugar or jelly
◗ Three glucose tablets (available without a prescription at most pharmacies)

If you experience symptoms of low blood sugar but can't check your blood sugar level right away, treat yourself as though you have hypoglycemia. In fact, you might want to carry at least one sugary item with you at all times. It's also a good idea to wear a bracelet that identifies you as someone who has diabetes.

Check your blood sugar level again 15 to 20 minutes later. If it's still too low, eat or drink something sugary. When you feel better, be sure to eat meals and snacks as usual.

When you meet with your doctor, mention any episodes of hypoglycemia. He or she will consider what triggered the hypoglycemia. If necessary, your doctor may change your diabetes treatment plan to prevent future problems with low blood sugar.

Prevention steps

The best way to manage hypoglycemia is to prevent it from occurring:

▶ If you have diabetes, follow the diabetes management plan you and your doctor have developed.
▶ If you don't have diabetes but have recurring episodes of hypoglycemia, eating frequent small meals throughout the day may keep your blood sugar levels from getting too low.

Overcoming barriers

Despite its advantages, many people with diabetes don't test their blood glucose as often as they should — or at all. Here are some common reasons why, along with some suggested solutions.

Cost

Many diabetes supply companies offer low-cost supplies. In addition, many diabetes drug companies have patient-assistance programs. If cost is a factor for you, talk with your doctor or diabetes educator and ask if there's a local or nationwide program that can help defray your expenses.

Limited access to health care

If getting to a medical center is a problem, check with your local, county or state health department about outreach health care services.

Lack of information and misperceptions

Some people are simply unaware of the benefits of blood glucose monitoring and believe there is nothing they can do to improve their disease. One of the best weapons in managing diabetes is education. Learn as much as you can about your disease.

Fear

If you fear the discomfort of pricking your finger, keep in mind that newer lancets are less painful.

Lifestyle issues

Even with a hectic or unconventional work schedule, you can find ways to build monitoring into your daily routine. Your doctor or diabetes educator can help with this.

Privacy issues

Testing is quick, and monitors are portable. You may be able to find a private place, such as a bathroom, to do your tests. But if you have to check your blood glucose in public, remember millions of people do it every day.

Chapter 3
Developing a Healthy-Eating Plan

Debunking the diabetes 'diet' 52

What's healthy eating? 53

Plan your meals 57

Watch your serving sizes 58

Size up your plate 60

Read food labels 61

Consider carb counting 62

The scoop on sugar 64

Using exchange lists 65

Keeping motivated 67

Recipes for good health 68

A visit with Sara Weigel

"Don't forget about consistency! We may choose the healthiest foods in the healthiest amounts, but skipping meals and erratic eating patterns may wreak havoc on blood sugar control and much-wanted weight loss."

Behavior and lifestyle changes are key to managing diabetes. In order to see changes in your health, you must make changes in some part of your everyday living. And nutrition is a great place to start!

Healthy eating for diabetes continues to evolve. Healthy eating in portioned amounts will always be fundamental to good overall health, but diabetes nutrition recommendations are driven by individual nutrition needs and preferences, too.

There are many reasons why nutrition for diabetes may look different from one person to the next. People may have different types of eating plans and patterns that are based on personal preferences, cultural beliefs as well as daily schedules and other medical issues.

Consider starting with the plate method. This consists of covering at least half of your plate with veggies, a quarter of the plate with lean protein, the remaining quarter of the plate with whole grains, starches, or beans and legumes, and adding a serving of milk or yogurt and fruit. Strive to choose the most heart-healthy options. Include regular physical activity as another way to assist in controlling your blood sugar and maintaining or losing weight.

There are typically three basic questions to think about if you're looking to improve your eating habits:

1. **How big is your portion?** A large portion of veggies is always a good idea, but typically a smaller portion of protein is recommended. Are your veggies taking up more room on the plate than your protein? Again, use the plate method as your guide.

2. **How is your food made?** Is it fried, grilled, baked? Choosing heart-healthy cooking techniques such as baking, grilling, boiling or broiling will continue to keep your food in its healthiest state without adding extra fat and calories.

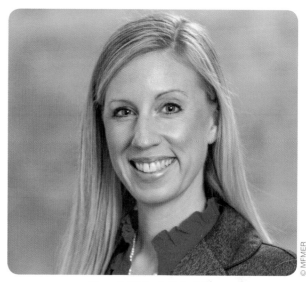

Sara E. Weigel, R.D., L.D.
Nutrition

3. **What do you put on your food?** Try to choose very small portions of added fats, and flavor with seasonings or spices instead of salt.

Don't forget about consistency! We may choose the healthiest foods in the healthiest amounts, but skipping meals and other erratic eating patterns may wreak havoc on your blood sugar control and any much-wanted weight loss.

Remember that eating should be enjoyed, not a chore. The best type of eating plan that you can follow is one that allows you to eat healthy, balanced meals that you enjoy.

It's recommended that you regularly visit with your diabetes care team. Because diabetes is a progressive disease, insulin and medications may be added or changed in order to keep your blood sugar under control. With a change in medication or insulin may come a change in nutrition recommendations.

Consider meeting with a registered dietitian to discuss how to incorporate healthy eating into your lifestyle as well as practical tools for achieving your goals such as glucose control, weight loss and improved nutrition.

Do the words *healthy eating* produce a twinge of fear? Some people may think, "Oh no, I'll never get to eat my favorite treats again!" But healthy eating isn't about deprivation or denial. It means enjoying great nutrition as well as great taste.

Healthy eating can mean updating your routine fare with delicious foods that you haven't tried before and experimenting with recipes to make them tasty as well as nutritious. A healthy diet is key to a healthy life, especially if you have diabetes or you're at risk.

Debunking the diabetes 'diet'

Contrary to popular myth, having diabetes doesn't mean that you have to start eating special foods or follow a complicated diet plan. For most people, eating well when you have diabetes simply translates into heart-healthy eating in portioned amounts.

This means choosing many plant-based foods such as vegetables, fruits and whole grains — and smaller servings of lean or low-fat animal foods, such as lean

cuts of meat and low-fat and fat-free dairy products. This kind of eating plan is naturally rich in nutrients and low in fat and calories. In fact, it's the same eating plan that all Americans should aim to follow.

Depending on the type of diabetes you have, your blood sugar (glucose) level, whether you need to lose weight and whether you have other health problems, you will need to tailor your eating plan somewhat to meet your personal needs. But even though the details may differ, the basics remain the same for everyone with diabetes. (See Healthy eating for all types of diabetes, next page).

What's healthy eating?

If you think that eating well means just counting calories or tallying fat grams, it's time to think about food in a different manner. Eating well means enjoying great taste as well as great nutrition.

Because your body is a complex machine, it needs a variety of foods to achieve a balanced mix of energy.

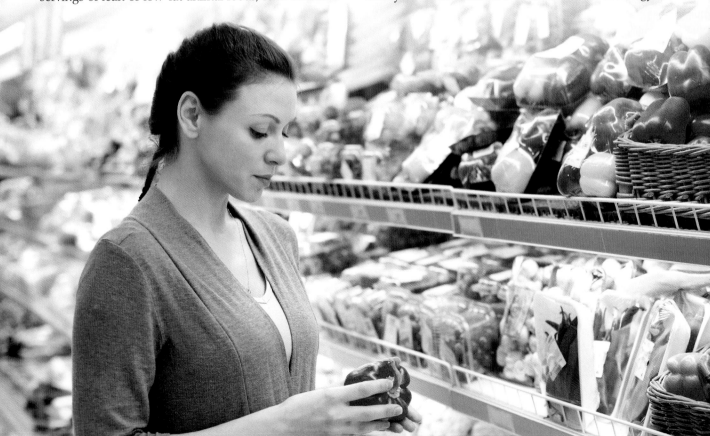

An eating plan that emphasizes a variety of vegetables, fruits and whole grains provides a rich supply of nutrients, fiber and other substances associated with better health. In addition, a variety of foods introduces you to many textures and flavors to increase eating pleasure.

By learning more about how your body uses the nutrients different foods provide, you'll better understand how eating well affects diabetes and your overall health.

Each day you want to eat a variety of foods that help you balance key nutrients. The three main nutrients that your body needs in large quantities (macronutrients) are carbohydrates, protein and fats. These macronutrients, when eaten in the right amounts, form the basis of a healthy-eating plan, for people with diabetes and for people without, alike.

Carbohydrates: The foundation

Carbohydrates (carbs) are your body's main energy source. During digestion, carbohydrates break down into glucose, or sugar — also known as energy for your body. Your brain, for example, uses glucose as its primary source of fuel.

Carbohydrate is the main macronutrient that raises blood sugar. But don't be alarmed — choosing the healthiest choices of carbohydrates in portioned amounts is key. Keeping the amount of carbohydrates you eat consistent throughout the day and day to day is a main way to keep your blood sugar under control.

It's typical for about half of your daily calories to come from carbohydrates. The number of servings depends on your calorie needs — ask your doctor or dietitian what's best for you.

Healthy eating for all types of diabetes

The main concepts of healthy eating for diabetes are similar whether you have prediabetes, type 1 or type 2 diabetes. They include these important steps:

▶ Adopting a heart-healthy eating plan
▶ Eating in portioned amounts
▶ Staying consistent with three meals a day at regular times
▶ Achieving and maintaining a healthy weight
▶ Limiting your intake of alcohol, sweets and sweetened beverages
▶ Following-up regularly with a dietitian and diabetes care team

However, one size doesn't fit all. The goals and specific nutrition suggestions for the different types of diabetes — as well as for your own individual circumstances — may vary:

Type	Goals	Nutrition suggestions
Prediabetes	Heart-healthy eating, physical activity, and weight loss or maintenance to keep blood sugars within normal ranges and prevent type 2 diabetes	Plate method of eating (see page 60) for balanced nutrition in portioned amounts
Type 2 diabetes	Heart-healthy eating, physical activity, weight loss or maintenance, as well as matching your diabetes treatment plan (oral medications, insulin) with your nutrition goals	Any or all: ▶ Plate method of eating for balanced nutrition in portioned amounts ▶ Carbohydrate counting (see page 62) ▶ Exchange system — a meal plan with specific portions of each food group (see page 65)
Type 1 diabetes	Heart-healthy eating and taking insulin to cover carbohydrate-containing foods	Carbohydrate counting

Carbohydrate myths and facts

Carbohydrates have gotten a bad reputation over the years. But the truth is, carbohydrates are good for your body when taken in moderation and as part of a healthy, balanced diet. Here's a look at the common myths and facts.

Myth: Carbohydrates are bad
Fact: Carbohydrates are needed to help provide your body, brain and nervous system energy to function. Carbohydrates are the body's main source of energy. They have important vitamins and minerals and are also your body's only source of dietary fiber.

Myth: Carbohydrates are only found in breads and sweets
Fact: Carbohydrates are included in many foods, such as fruits and fruit juices; milk and yogurt; grains, breads and pasta; starchy vegetables such as corn and potatoes; and sweets.

Myth: Carbohydrates cause weight gain
Fact: Carbohydrates, just like fat and protein, provide your body with calories. If too many calories are eaten, no matter what the food, the extra calories are stored as fat.

To help control your glucose level, eat about the same amount of carbohydrates at each of three meals daily.

Protein: The building block

Your body uses protein for the development and maintenance of your muscles and organs. Foods high in protein include meat, poultry, eggs, cheese, fish, legumes, and nuts, seeds and nut butters. If you eat more protein than you need — which many people do — your body stores these extra calories as fat.

Select proteins that are lower in fat, such as fish, poultry without skin, lean meats, and low-fat or fat-free cheese. Whether or not you're a vegetarian, plant sources of protein, such as legumes (beans, dried peas and lentils) and products made from soy (miso, tempeh, tofu, soy milk and soy cheese), can replace meat and dairy products. These foods are also low in fat and cholesterol. Consider this a chance to try something new.

Fats: The calorie heavyweights

Fats are the most concentrated source of food energy. Fat is essential to the life and function of your cells. It's when you eat too much fat — and the wrong kinds — that health problems occur.

Not all fats are created equal. Plus they're high in calories, so it's important to limit total fat consumption to help control your weight, blood sugar and blood cholesterol.

To limit the amount of fat you eat, follow these tips:

- Buy lean cuts of meat and trim off the excess fat. Also eat smaller amounts.
- Remove the skin from poultry before cooking.
- Marinate meats and use herbs and spices to keep them tender, moist and give them flavor.
- Avoid fried foods. Instead, bake, steam, grill, broil or roast meat and vegetables.
- Choose fat-free or low-fat dairy products, salad dressings and spreads.
- Use canola or olive oil (in small amounts) for cooking and salads.
- Season vegetables with lemon, lime or herbs rather than butter or oil.
- Replace some of the shortening in baked goods with applesauce or prune puree.

Fats: The good and the bad

As you read labels, look for products that contain monounsaturated fats with little or no saturated and trans fats. Remember that all fats are high in calories.

Monounsaturated fats ("good fats") help lower total and low-density lipoprotein (LDL, or "bad") cholesterol. They're found mainly in olive, canola and peanut oils, as well as most nuts and avocados.

Polyunsaturated fats help lower total and LDL cholesterol. They're found mainly in vegetable oils such as safflower, corn, sunflower, soy and cottonseed.

Saturated fats raise total and LDL cholesterol, increasing your risk of heart disease. They're found mainly in red meats, most whole-fat dairy products (including butter), egg yolks, chocolate (cocoa butter), as well as coconut, palm and other tropical oils.

Trans fats, also called partially hydrogenated vegetable oil, raise LDL cholesterol, increasing your risk of heart disease. They're found mainly in stick margarine and shortening and the products made from them — cookies, pastry, other baked goods, most crackers, candies, snack foods and french fries.

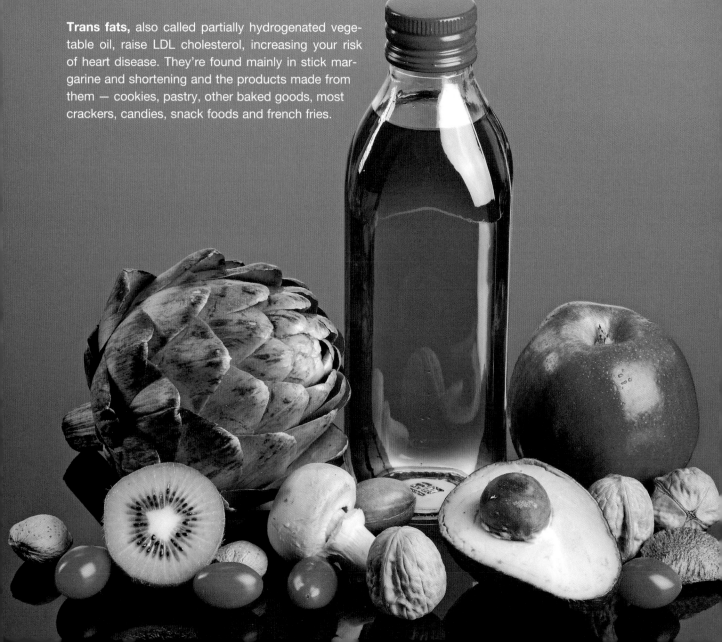

Keep an eye on saturated fat and cholesterol

Because diabetes puts you at increased risk of heart disease and stroke, it's also important that you limit your intake of saturated fat and cholesterol. Saturated fat elevates your blood cholesterol levels. When there's too much cholesterol in your blood, you may develop fatty deposits in your blood vessels. Eventually, these deposits make it difficult for blood to flow through your arteries.

The most concentrated sources of saturated fat and cholesterol include high-fat animal products such as organ meats and processed meats, egg yolks and high-fat dairy products (including whole milk, cream, ice cream and full-fat cheese). Instead, use lean cuts of meat, egg substitutes, and low-fat or fat-free milk products whenever possible.

Don't forget your omega-3s

Eating fish that is rich in omega-3 fatty acids can help protect against coronary artery disease. Fish is also a good alternative to high-fat meats.

Fish high in omega-3 fats include anchovies, bass (striped, sea and freshwater), bluefish, herring, salmon, sardines, trout (rainbow and lake) and tuna (especially white, albacore and bluefin), among others.*

Eating at least two 3-ounce servings of these types of fish every week is recommended.

*The Food and Drug Administration advises pregnant women, nursing mothers and children to eat up to 12 ounces of fish a week. Don't eat king mackerel, shark, swordfish or tilefish because these types of fish have higher amounts of mercury. Limit albacore tuna and tuna steaks to no more than 6 ounces a week.

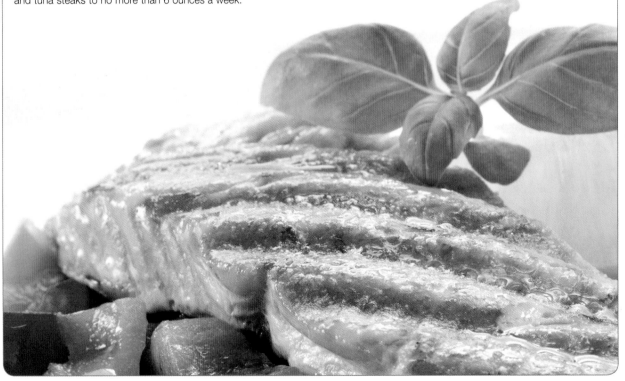

Plan your meals

A meal plan is simply an eating guide with two key points:

1. It helps establish a routine for eating meals at regular times every day.
2. It guides you in choosing the healthiest foods in the right amounts at each meal.

When you're first diagnosed with diabetes, ask your doctor to refer you to a dietitian. Eating at irregular times, overeating or making poor food choices can contribute to high blood glucose. A doctor or dietitian can provide you with tips to improve your eating habits.

Some people may need to follow a more deliberate plan, eating only the recommended number of servings from each food group every day, based on their individual calorie needs. A registered dietitian can help you with a plan to improve eating habits and better manage your diabetes.

Working with a dietitian

Understanding the healthiest food choices, how much to eat and how those food choices affect your blood glucose level can be a complex task. A registered dietitian can help you make sense of all this information and put together a plan that's easy to follow and that fits your health goals, food tastes, family or cultural traditions, and lifestyle.

At the first meeting, your dietitian will likely ask you about your weight history and your eating habits — what you like to eat, how much you generally eat, as well as when and what time of day you have meals and snacks.

You'll also likely discuss your diabetes treatment goals, what medications you take, any special health considerations, your physical activity level, your work schedule and your calorie needs, and whether you're trying to lose weight.

Together you and your dietitian will figure out what's practical and achievable for you and what's not. Then you'll both decide on the best meal-planning tool to help you control your diabetes. The most common tools for planning meals are the plate method, carbohydrate counting and exchange lists.

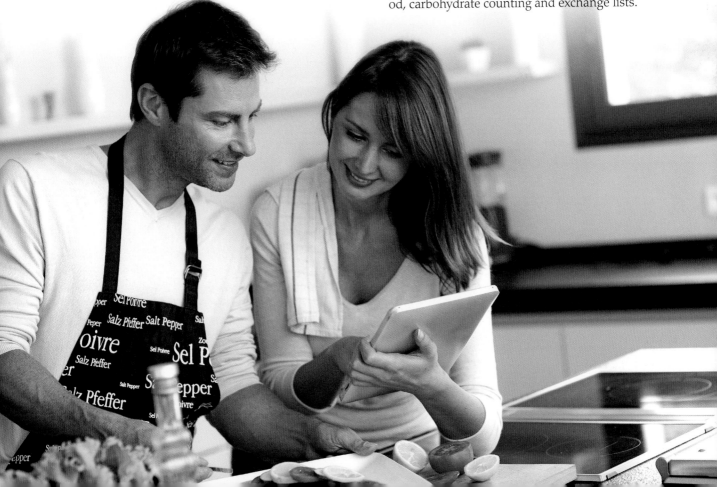

Consistency is key

If you're consistent in your eating habits, it can help control your blood glucose levels. Every day try to eat:

▶ At about the same time
▶ The same number of meals and about the same amount of food

Stick to your routine. It's more difficult to control your blood glucose if you eat a small lunch and a large evening meal the same day. And the more you vary the amount of carbohydrates that you eat meal to meal or day to day, the harder it is to control your blood glucose.

Eating at regularly spaced intervals — meals spaced about four to five hours apart — reduces large variations in blood glucose and also allows for adequate digestion and metabolism of food.

Look for variety

Aim for a wide mix of foods to help you meet your nutritional goals. Your dietitian can help you plan a program that includes a healthy variety of foods.

This doesn't mean that you have to seek out unusual "diet foods." Instead focus on eating more vegetables, fruits, whole grains, lean meats and low-fat dairy prod-

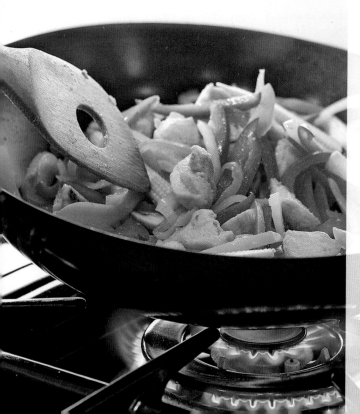

ucts. And it doesn't mean preparing dishes that are complicated or expensive. Some of the world's most tempting dishes are built around the season's best produce, prepared simply to bring out the fullest flavors.

People who regularly enjoy meals made with a variety of healthy ingredients reduce their risk of developing diabetes or complications from the disease. What's more, they also reduce their risk of developing many other diseases, including heart disease, many kinds of cancer, digestive disorders, age-related vision loss and osteoporosis.

Watch your serving sizes

A serving isn't the amount of food you choose to eat or the amount that's put on your plate. This is called a portion. Rather, a serving is a specific amount of food, defined by standard measurements, such as cups, ounces or pieces.

Pay close attention to serving sizes. With the trend toward supersizing, mega-buffets and huge portions in restaurants, you may not have an accurate idea of what a regular serving size is.

At first, the serving sizes may seem small. For example, 3 cups of popcorn (low-fat microwave or popped with no fat added) is one serving. This amount may hardly make a dent in the large bucket you're used to getting at the movies.

Your ability to monitor the number of servings you eat at meals is key to meeting your daily nutritional goals.

Keeping all of the food groups and measurements straight may seem overwhelming. Don't panic! Serving sizes aren't as complex as they may seem. You don't need to have the entire list memorized in your head. Start with the foods that you eat most frequently. You'll be surprised at how quickly you'll retain this knowledge. However, it does take some practice.

Sometimes just being aware of the serving size on a nutrition label will help guide you in the right amount to eat.

Sizing up a serving

An important part of eating healthy is understanding how much of a particular food makes up a serving. Many people envision servings to be larger than they are, and they eat more than they should. This page provides some visual clues to help you gauge general serving sizes.

Vegetables	Visual cue	
1 cup broccoli 2 cups raw, leafy greens	1 baseball 2 baseballs	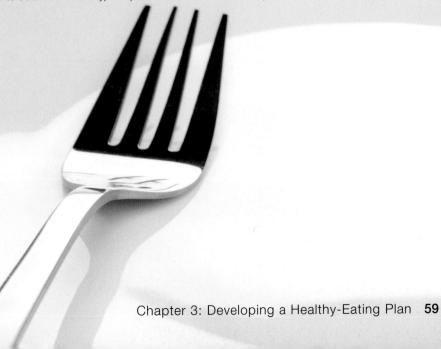
Fruits*	**Visual cue**	
½ cup sliced fruit 1 small apple or medium orange	Tennis ball	
Starch (carbohydrates)	**Visual cue**	
½ cup pasta, rice or dried cereal ½ bagel 1 slice whole-grain bread	Hockey puck	
Protein and dairy* †	**Visual cue**	
2½ ounces chicken or fish 1½ ounces beef 1½ ounces beef	Deck of cards ½ deck of cards 4 dice	
Fats	**Visual cue**	
1½ teaspoons peanut butter 1 teaspoon butter or margarine	2 dice 1 die	

*Fruits, milk and yogurt are also sources of carbohydrate that can affect blood sugar.
†There are many types of meal-planning tools. The Mayo Clinic Healthy Weight Pyramid groups meats and milk products together, whereas the American Diabetes Association and the Academy of Nutrition and Dietetics separate meats and milk products in their diabetes exchange lists. Work with your health care provider to determine which type of plan will be most effective for you.

Size up your plate

Consistent, balanced meals are an important aspect of blood sugar control. But this doesn't have to require careful calculations.

Instead, consider using the plate method — a simple but effective way to help you know how much to eat at mealtime. Follow these steps to help you choose the right portions.

1. Try to fill half your plate with nonstarchy vegetables. These include all vegetables except potatoes, beans and lentils, corn, peas, or winter squash. Enjoy nonstarchy vegetables often and make them the largest part of your plate. Flavor vegetables with herbs and spices rather than with salt, fats or oils.

2. Keep the portion of meat and meat substitutes to no more than one-quarter of your plate (about the size of a deck of cards). Meat includes beef, pork, fish, poultry and other animal proteins such as eggs. Meat substitutes include cheese, peanut butter, nuts, seeds and tofu. Bake, broil, boil or grill these foods. Avoid adding extra fats or frying. These are high-fat sources of protein, so limit your portions.

3. Use the remainder of your plate for a carbohydrate. Remember that carbohydrate choices can be fruits or milk and yogurt.

In addition, try to limit the amount of fat you add to your cooking and to your meal. Choose healthier fat options, such as olive, canola and peanut oils. If you have questions, talk to your doctor or dietitian.

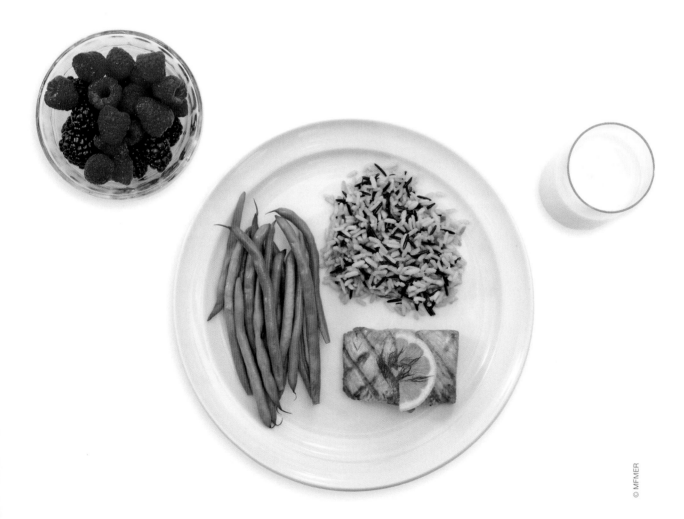

© MFMER

Read food labels

Food labels can be an essential tool for diabetes meal planning. Here are some tips for comparing food labels.

Do the math

The serving sizes listed on food labels may be different from the amounts you're used to eating. If you eat twice the serving size as listed on the label, you also double the calories, fat, carbohydrate and sodium.

Control calories

Calories can add up fast. It's important to be aware of the amount of calories you're eating, especially if you're trying to lose weight. Although some foods may be fat-free or low carb, this doesn't mean they're calorie-free. Think of calories like a daily allowance of money. If the goal is to maintain your weight, it's best to stay within your budgeted amount of calories most of the time. A dietitian can help you determine the right amount of calories for your personal goal, whether it's weight loss or weight maintenance.

Consider carbs in context

Look at the grams of total carbohydrate — which includes sugar, complex carbohydrate and fiber — rather than only the grams of sugar. If you zero in on only the sugar content, you could miss out on nutritious foods that contain natural sugar, such as fruit, yogurt and milk. And you might overdo foods with no natural or added sugar but plenty of carbohydrate, such as certain cereals and grains.

The goal is not to eat as few carbohydrates as you can, but rather to choose to the healthiest carbohydrate in consistent amounts from meal to meal. Ask your dietitian how many carbohydrates he or she would recommend for you at meals.

Put sugar-free products in their place

Products labeled "sugar-free" are often touted as the best choice for people with diabetes. However, sugar-free doesn't mean carbohydrate-free. When choosing between standard products and their sugar-free counterparts, don't assume sugar-free is better. Compare the food labels side by side.

If the sugar-free product has noticeably fewer carbohydrates, it might be the better choice. But if there's little difference in carbohydrates, fat and calories between the two foods, let taste — or price — be your guide.

The same caveat applies to products sporting a "no sugar added" label. Although these foods don't contain high-sugar ingredients and no sugar is added during processing or packaging, foods without added sugar may still be high in carbohydrates.

Scan the list of ingredients

Keep an eye out for heart-healthy ingredients such as whole-wheat flour, soy and oats. Monounsaturated fats — such as olive, canola or peanut oils — promote heart health, too. Likewise, use food labels to detect unhealthy ingredients, such as hydrogenated or partially hydrogenated oil.

Keep in mind that ingredients are listed in descending order by weight. The main ingredient is listed first, followed by other ingredients used in lesser amounts. For example, if you're looking for a whole-grain product, make sure a whole grain is listed as the first ingredient.

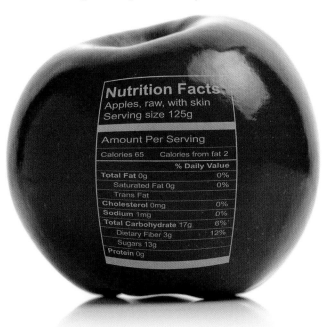

Nutrition Facts
Apples, raw, with skin
Serving size 125g

Amount Per Serving

Calories 65   Calories from fat 2

% Daily Value

Total Fat 0g   0%
  Saturated Fat 0g   0%
  Trans Fat
Cholesterol 0mg   0%
Sodium 1mg   0%
Total Carbohydrate 17g   6%
  Dietary Fiber 3g   12%
  Sugars 13g
Protein 0g

Consider carb counting

Carbohydrate counting is a method of controlling the amount of carbohydrates you eat at meals and snacks. This is because carbohydrates have the greatest impact on your blood glucose.

It's the balance between the carbohydrates you eat and insulin that determines how much your blood glucose levels rise after you eat. With the right balance of carbohydrates and insulin, your blood glucose level will usually come back into goal range.

Carb counting and diabetes

Some people with diabetes — especially those who take diabetes medications or insulin — use carbohydrate counting as a meal-planning tool. They count the amount of carbohydrates in each meal or snack. This helps keep their blood glucose from going too high or too low throughout the day.

However, carbohydrate counting doesn't mean that you can go overboard on foods that are low in or free of carbohydrates, such as meat and fats. These foods are high in calories.

Too many calories and too much fat and cholesterol over the long term increase your risk of weight gain, heart disease, stroke and other diseases, as well as make it difficult to control your blood sugar.

Understand the terms

If you're counting carbs, be aware that the term *net carbohydrates* or *net carbs* on product labels can be misleading. These marketing terms aren't approved by the Food and Drug Administration (FDA), so if you use the net carb number on the label you may not accurately be counting your carbohydrates. And if you're on insulin, you could underestimate how much you need. Work with your dietitian to learn how to count carbs properly to meet your specific needs.

Be consistent

With carb counting, and diabetes in general, consistency is very important. Large variations in your carbohydrate intake throughout the day — such as skipping meals and then eating a huge meal — can cause blood glucose levels to go too high or too low.

Also, it's important not to confuse carb counting with fad-diet terminology. A low-carb diet is not the same as carb counting.

How to count carbs

You may be thinking that carb counting sounds like a lot of work. Relax. Your dietitian will determine how many carbs you should aim for at meals.

? **Is the glycemic index another good tool for planning meals?**

The glycemic index (GI) ranks carbohydrate-containing foods based on their effect on blood glucose levels. High-index foods are associated with greater increases in blood glucose than are low-index foods. But low-index foods aren't necessarily healthier. Foods that are high in fat tend to have lower GI values than do some healthy foods.

Using the GI for meal planning is a fairly complicated process. Many factors affect the GI value of a specific food, such as how the food was prepared and what you eat with it. Also, the GI value for some foods isn't known. Another meal-planning tool is the glycemic load, which multiplies the GI of a food by the amount of total carbohydrates in a serving. For example, eating small amounts of a food with a high glycemic load may have less impact on blood glucose.

Talk with a registered dietitian if you have questions. Currently there isn't enough evidence of benefits to recommend using GI diets as your main strategy in meal planning.

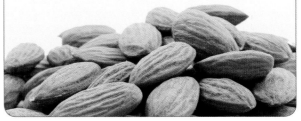

You also don't have to memorize how many carbs are in a glass of milk, a cookie or a piece of fruit. Instead, you can purchase books or use online resources or mobile programs (apps) that list carb counts for thousands of foods, and most packaged foods are required to list their carb counts right on the label.

Here are a few tips to get you started:

- Begin with the Nutrition Facts label that's on most packaged foods. The most important information you need for carb counting is the "Serving Size" and the "Total Carbohydrate." Start with the serving size. For example, one serving of chili equals 1 cup, and 1 cup of chili contains 22 grams (g) of carbohydrates.
- Next, guess how much you'll probably eat. Is it about 1 cup, or more like 2 cups? Then do the math. Two cups have 44 g of carbohydrates.
- Now think about the other foods you're going to eat with your chili. Crackers and a piece of fruit? There are carbs in these foods, too. About how much will you eat, and what's the total carb count?
- If you're eating fresh foods that don't come packaged, you can usually get the carb information in books or online.

What about recipes?

You may be thinking: "What about recipes? How do I count the carbs in homemade foods? Do I have to add together the carbohydrate amounts for each separate ingredient?"

Well, for some foods, that may be the easiest way to do it. Take a tuna salad sandwich, for example. It includes two slices of bread, half a can of tuna and a couple of tablespoons of mayonnaise. Check the serving sizes and carb counts for the bread, tuna and mayonnaise. In this case, the tuna and mayo have minimal carbs, so you only need to count the bread.

At first, you may have to measure your foods to get a sense of how much you use. But after a while, you'll be able to "eyeball" the serving sizes pretty well.

Now, what about more-complicated foods, such as lasagna? Well, you can get books that list approximate carb counts for homemade foods. This would be a good starting point. Or you can get cookbooks, software and mobile apps that will give you carb counts for all kinds of foods.

Some software will calculate nutrition facts after you add or subtract ingredients from recipes, or even enter your own recipes.

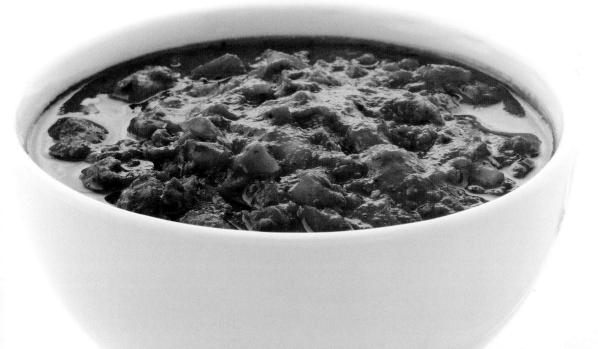

The scoop on sugar

For years, people with diabetes were warned to avoid sweets and sugars. But what researchers understand about diabetes nutrition has changed — and so has the advice on sweets.

It was once assumed that honey, candy and other sweets would raise your blood sugar level faster and higher than fruits, vegetables or foods containing complex carbohydrates. But many studies have shown this isn't true, as long as the sweets are eaten with a meal and balanced with other foods. Although different types of sweets can affect your blood sugar level differently, it's the total amount of carbohydrate that counts the most.

Of course, it's still best to consider sweets only a small part of your overall diet. Candy, cookies and other sweets have little nutritional value and are often high in fat and calories. These foods aren't the best choices for anyone, regardless of diabetes status.

'Have your cake and eat it too'

Sweets count as carbohydrates in your meal plan. The trick is substituting small portions of sweets for other carbohydrates — such as bread, tortillas, rice, crackers, cereal, fruit, milk or yogurt — in your meals. To allow room for sweets as part of a meal, you have two options:

▶ Replace some of the carbohydrates in your meal with a sweet.
▶ Swap a carb-containing food in your meal for something with fewer carbohydrates.

Let's say your typical lunch is a turkey sandwich with a glass of skim milk and a piece of fresh fruit. If you'd like a cookie with your meal, look for ways to keep the total carbohydrate count in the meal the same. Trade your usual bread for low-calorie bread with fewer carbohydrates or eat an open-faced sandwich with only one slice of bread. Then when you add a cookie, the total carbohydrate count stays the same.

To make sure you're making even trades, read food labels carefully. Look for the total carbohydrate in each food, which tells you how much carbohydrate is in one serving.

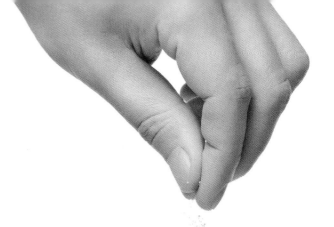

Consider sugar substitutes

Artificial sweeteners offer the sweetness of sugar without the calories. Artificial sweeteners may help you reduce calories and total carbohydrates and stick to a healthy plan — especially when used instead of sugar in coffee and tea, on cereal, or in baked goods. In fact, artificial sweeteners, by themselves, are considered "free foods" because they contain very few calories and don't increase blood sugar significantly.

Examples of artificial sweeteners include:

▶ Acesulfame potassium (Sweet One, Sunett)
▶ Aspartame (Equal, NutraSweet)
▶ Saccharin (SugarTwin, Sweet'N Low)
▶ Sucralose (Splenda)

But artificial sweeteners don't necessarily offer a free pass for sweets. Many products made with artificial sweeteners, such as baked goods and artificially sweetened yogurt, still contain calories and carbohydrates that can affect your blood sugar level.

The same goes for sugar alcohols, another type of reduced-calorie sweetener often used in sugar-free candies and desserts. Check product labels for words such as *sorbitol*, *maltitol*, *mannitol*, *xylitol* and *lactitol*.

Although sugar alcohols are lower in calories than is regular sugar, sugar-free foods containing sugar alcohols still have calories. And in some people, sugar alcohols can cause diarrhea, gas and bloating.

A change in taste

Don't be surprised if your tastes change as you adopt healthier eating habits. Food that you once loved may seem too sweet — and healthy substitutes may become your new idea of delicious.

Using exchange lists

Meal plans that include exchanges are one type of tool you might consider using to control your blood sugar and weight while striving to get balanced nutrients.

In the exchange system, foods are grouped into basic types — such as starches, fruits, milk and milk products, and meat and meat substitutes. The foods within each group contain about the same amount of calories, carbohydrates and other nutrients.

That means you can exchange, or trade, foods within a group because they're similar in nutrient content and the manner in which they affect your blood sugar.

An exchange is basically one serving within a group. One starch exchange, for instance, might be half of a medium baked potato (3 ounces) or ⅓ cup of baked beans or ½ cup of corn.

Your dietitian may recommend a certain number of daily exchanges from each food group based on your personal needs and preferences. Together you'll decide the best way to spread the exchanges throughout the day.

Exchange lists, which are developed by the American Diabetes Association and the Academy of Nutrition and Dietetics, help ensure variety in your meal plan as well as the proper serving sizes to help keep your blood sugar level within your target range.

Food categories

In the exchange system, foods are grouped into these main categories:

▶ Starches
▶ Nonstarchy vegetables
▶ Fruits
▶ Milk and milk products
▶ Meat and meat substitutes
▶ Sweets and other carbohydrates
▶ Fats

The exchange system also includes information on determining exchanges when eating or drinking:

▶ Combination foods
▶ Fast foods
▶ Alcohol

Another category in the exchange system is called free foods. A free food is a food or drink that has fewer than 20 calories or no more than 5 grams of carbohydrate per serving.

Getting on the exchange

Talk to your doctor or dietitian about how using exchange lists might help improve your eating habits and get your diabetes under better control.

? Can I eat or drink foods or beverages with artificial sweeteners in unlimited amounts?

Most beverages and some hard candies that contain artificial sweeteners have almost no calories, and they don't count as a carbohydrate, a fat or any other exchange. Examples include:

▶ Acesulfame potassium (Sweet One, Sunett)
▶ Aspartame (Equal, NutraSweet)
▶ Saccharin (SugarTwin, Sweet'N Low)
▶ Sucralose (Splenda)

Keep in mind that many foods labeled as diet, dietetic or sugar-free (such as sugar-free candies) contain sweeteners with calories and carbohydrates that may affect your glucose level. Check product labels for words such as *sorbitol*, *mannitol*, *xylitol*, *lactitol* and *maltitol*, which are sugar alcohols.

Although sugar alcohols are lower in calories than sugar, don't eat unlimited quantities of sugar-free foods because other ingredients in these foods contribute calories. And in some people, sugar alcohols can cause diarrhea, gas and bloating.

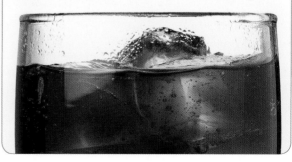

Diabetes and alcohol: Do they mix?

Many people with diabetes wonder if it's OK to drink alcohol. The best advice is to ask your doctor about appropriate alcohol intake for your specific situation. If you're having trouble controlling your blood glucose or if you have high levels of triglycerides — a type of blood fat — you may be advised to avoid alcohol. But a light to moderate amount may be fine if your diabetes is well-controlled and it doesn't interfere with your medication.

If you choose to drink alcohol, do so in moderation. For healthy adults, that means up to one drink a day for women of all ages and men older than age 65, and up to two drinks a day for men age 65 and younger. One drink equals one 12-ounce can of regular beer (about 150 calories), one 5-ounce glass of wine (about 100 calories) or one 1½-ounce shot glass of hard liquor (about 100 calories).

Always drink alcohol with a meal or with food. Never drink on an empty stomach because of the risk of low blood glucose. Remember, high-calorie beverages (especially mixed drinks that include sugary sodas and juices) can raise blood glucose and contribute to weight gain.

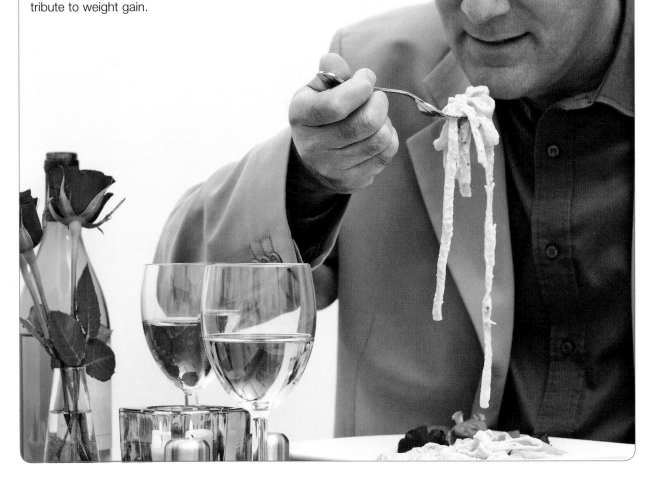

Keeping motivated

Sticking to a healthy-eating plan is one of the most challenging aspects of living with diabetes. The key is to find ways to keep motivated and overcome hurdles.

Financial concerns

Buying lots of fresh fruits and vegetables can be expensive. But keep in mind that you're probably buying fewer less-nutritious foods, such as chips and sweets, which also can be costly. You also save money if you buy less meat. And frozen and canned fruits (without added sugar) and vegetables (without added salt and fat) are less expensive, healthy options that don't spoil as quickly as fresh produce.

Cultural barriers

Food is an expression of culture. But all cuisine can be prepared in healthier ways. You can find cookbooks for people with diabetes that focus on foods from different cultures, with plenty of ideas for making recipes healthier.

Family and social situations

Sometimes family members and friends may not understand why you're making changes to your meals — and to theirs. Discuss your diabetes treatment goals with family and friends and ask them for their support. The changes you're making will help keep you and your family healthy.

If family and friends seem offended if you say no to their special dishes, enlist their aid to help make that special recipe a healthy option. Ask your dietitian for recipe suggestions so that you can include family favorites in your meal plan.

If you're going to attend a special gathering where you don't know the people well, before you arrive think through what you'll eat and drink once you get there. You might also consider bringing along your own healthy snacks.

Rewards of staying on plan

Motivation to stick with your healthy-eating plan will improve as you begin to experience the benefits of your hard work:

- You'll experience fewer episodes of high and low blood glucose.
- You'll be better able to control your weight.
- You'll feel better and have more energy.
- You'll have greater control over your diabetes.

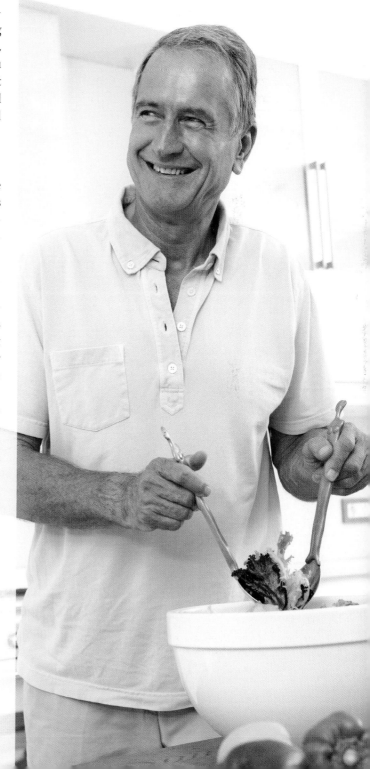

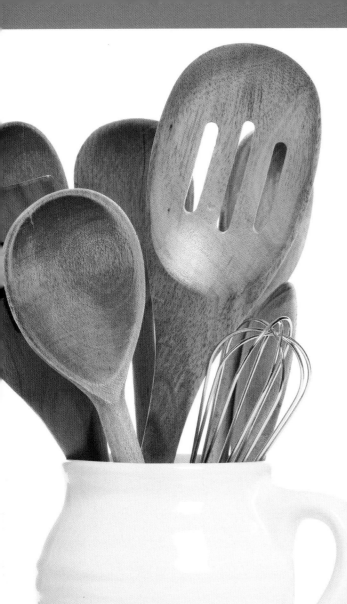

Recipes
for good health

The decisions you make each day about selecting and preparing food affect how you feel today and how well you'll live in the years ahead.

How do you eat well? It begins with enjoying a variety of foods that can help keep you healthy. If you have diabetes, eating well will help keep your blood glucose in check, possibly preventing you from having to take medication or reducing the amount that you need to take.

The recipes that follow show how easy and enjoyable eating well can be.

Baked Chicken With Pears
Serves 8

Ingredients
8 4-oz. boneless, skinless chicken breasts
1 tsp. tarragon
1 tbsp. olive oil (divided)
4 medium sweet onions, thinly sliced
4 pears, seeds removed and thinly sliced
1 c. low-fat feta cheese crumbles

Preparation
1. Preheat oven to 375 F.
2. Rub each chicken breast with tarragon.
3. In a large, ovenproof skillet heat ½ tablespoon olive oil and cook breasts 2 to 3 minutes per side until lightly golden. Add remaining oil and sliced onion and continue to cook until onions are translucent.
4. Lightly cover the skillet with foil. Place skillet in oven and bake chicken and onions about 15 minutes. Chicken breast should reach 165 F when tested with a meat thermometer. Remove from oven. Let rest (still covered) about 5 minutes before serving.
5. Plate chicken as follows: Make a bed of cooked onion, place chicken on top. Arrange pear slices on and around chicken breast. Sprinkle each with 2 tablespoons feta. Serve.

Per serving
Calories - 259
Total fat - 3 g
Saturated fat - < 1 g
Monounsaturated fat - 1.6 g
Cholesterol - 67 mg
Sodium - 258 mg
Carbohydrate - 26 g
Fiber - 4 g
Protein - 32 g

Exchange list servings
Fruits - 1
Nonstarchy vegetables - 2
Meat and meat substitutes - 3

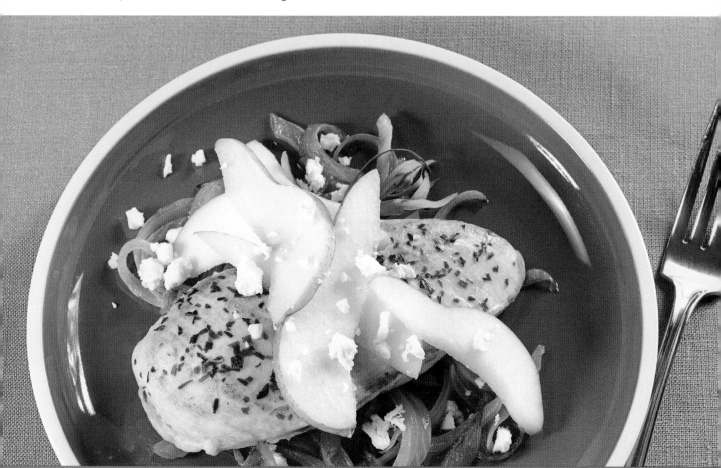

Brown Rice With Vegetables
Serves 8

Ingredients
1 c. brown rice, uncooked
1 tbsp. oil
2 c. reduced-sodium chicken broth (or water)
4 scallions (green onions including tops)
2 c. total – red, green or yellow bell peppers, celery, mushrooms, asparagus, pea pods or carrots
2 tbsp. lemon juice
Optional: ground black pepper, chopped fresh parsley

Preparation
1. In a large saucepan, over medium heat, sauté the rice in oil for about 2 minutes stirring frequently. Reduce heat, add broth and simmer covered without stirring or opening the lid for about 30 minutes.
2. In the meantime, chop scallions including green tops into small pieces. Do the same with your choice of vegetables.
3. When rice has cooked 30 minutes, add the vegetables and lemon juice. Stir well to combine. Cover pan and continue to cook over medium heat until rice is tender but still has some texture (about 10 to 15 minutes more).
4. Season with black pepper and top with chopped fresh parsley (if desired) and serve.

Per serving
Calories - 123
Total fat - 2 g
Saturated fat - 0.5 g
Monounsaturated fat - 1.5 g
Cholesterol - 1 mg
Sodium - 44 mg
Carbohydrate - 21 g
Fiber - 2 g
Protein - 3 g

Exchange list servings
Starches - 1
Nonstarchy vegetables - 1
Fats - ½

Spring Greens With Acorn Squash
Serves 4

Ingredients
2 acorn squash (about 2 lbs. total)
2 tbsp. brown sugar
1 tbsp. trans fat-free margarine or olive oil
4 c. leaf lettuce (red-leaf, Boston, bibb or a mixture)
2 tbsp. sunflower seeds
4 tsp. honey

Preparation
1. Pierce the squash several times with a sharp knife to let the steam escape during cooking.
2. Microwave each squash on high until tender, about 5 minutes. Turn the squash after 3 minutes to ensure even cooking.
3. Place the squash on a cutting board and cut in half. Scrape out and discard the seeds.
4. Remove the pulp of the squash and put into a mixing bowl. Repeat with the second squash. There should be about 2 cups of pulp.
5. Sprinkle squash with the brown sugar and add the margarine. Mix until smooth. Set aside to cool slightly.
6. Divide the lettuce onto 4 salad plates. Top each with ½ cup of the squash mixture, ½ tablespoon sunflower seeds and 1 teaspoon honey. Serve immediately.

Per serving
Calories - 97
Total fat - 5 g
Saturated fat - 1 g
Monounsaturated fat - 2 g
Cholesterol - 0 mg
Sodium - 54 mg
Carbohydrate - 35 g
Fiber - 4 g
Protein - 3 g

Exchange list servings
Starches - 1
Sweets and other carbohydrates - 1
Fats - 1

Blueberry and Lemon Cream Parfait
Serves 4

Ingredients
6 oz. low-fat vanilla yogurt sweetened with low-calorie sweetener
4 oz. fat-free cream cheese
1 tsp. honey
2 tsp. freshly grated lemon zest
3 c. fresh blueberries, rinsed and drained well

Preparation
1. Drain liquid from the yogurt. In a medium bowl, combine the yogurt, cream cheese and honey. Use an electric mixer to beat at high speed until the yogurt mixture is light and creamy.
2. Stir the lemon zest into the mixture.
3. Layer the lemon cream and blueberries in dessert dishes. If not serving immediately, cover and refrigerate.

Per serving
Calories - 129
Total fat - 1 g
Saturated fat - trace
Monounsaturated fat - trace
Cholesterol - 4 mg
Sodium - 225 mg
Carbohydrate - 23 g
Fiber - 3 g
Protein - 7 g

Exchange list servings
Fruits - 1
Milk and milk products - ½

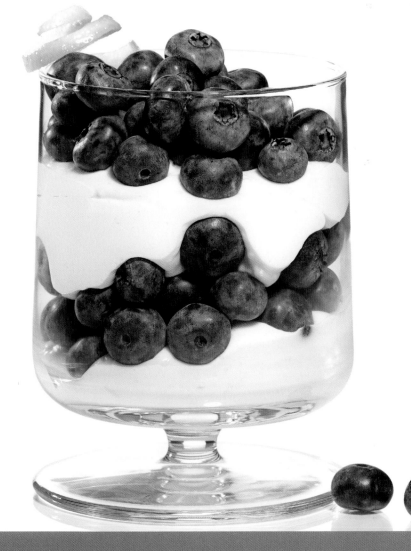

Roasted Potatoes
Serves 4

Ingredients
1 lb. large red or white potatoes with skins, cut into wedges ¼-inch thick
1 tbsp. olive oil
1 tsp. rosemary or oregano

Preparation
1. Preheat oven to 400 F.
2. Lightly coat a baking sheet with cooking spray.
3. Soak the potato wedges in ice water for 5 minutes. Drain the potatoes and rinse thoroughly under cold water. Press between paper towels to dry.
4. Transfer potatoes to a large bowl, pour the olive oil over the potatoes and toss to coat evenly.
5. Arrange the potatoes in a single layer on the prepared baking sheet.
6. Bake for 15 minutes. Turn the potatoes over and bake another 5 minutes. Sprinkle the herbs over the potatoes. Return the potatoes to the oven and bake until they're brown and crispy, about 5 minutes. Serve immediately.

Per serving
Calories - 116
Total fat - 4 g
Saturated fat - 0.5 g
Monounsaturated fat - 2 g
Cholesterol - 0 mg
Sodium - 20 mg
Carbohydrate - 18 g
Fiber - 2 g
Protein - 2 g

Exchange list servings
Starches - 1
Fats - 1

Grapes and Walnuts With Lemon Sour Cream Sauce
Serves 6

Ingredients
½ c. fat-free sour cream
2 tbsp. powdered sugar
½ tsp. lemon zest
½ tsp. lemon juice
⅛ tsp. vanilla extract
1½ c. red seedless grapes
1½ c. green seedless grapes
3 tbsp. chopped walnuts

Preparation
1. In a small bowl, combine sour cream, powdered sugar, lemon zest, lemon juice and vanilla. Whisk to mix evenly.
2. Cover and chill for several hours.
3. Divide grapes equally among 6 stemmed dessert glasses or bowls. Add 2 tablespoons of the lemon topping to each dish. Sprinkle each serving with ½ tablespoon of chopped walnuts. Serve immediately.

Per serving
Calories - 98
Total fat - 2 g
Saturated fat - trace
Monounsaturated fat - 0.5 g
Cholesterol - 0 mg
Sodium - 38 mg
Carbohydrate - 18 g
Fiber - 1 g
Protein - 2 g

Exchange list servings
Fruits - 1
Sweets - ½

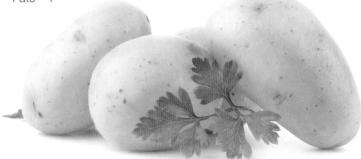

Seafood Kebab
Serves 6

Ingredients
1 lb. shrimp
1 lb. sea scallops
Juice from 1 lemon
2 tbsp. olive oil
1 garlic clove, minced
2 tbsp. chopped fresh cilantro

Preparation
1. Peel and devein shrimp, leaving tail on. Rinse and pat dry with paper towel. Rinse and pat scallops dry. Place shrimp and scallops into glass bowl. Add remaining ingredients. Toss well and marinate in refrigerator for at least 30 minutes.
2. Spray broiler pan or grate with cooking spray. Preheat broiler or grill. Alternate shrimp and scallops on skewers. Place under broiler or onto grill for several minutes. Brush with any marinade while grilling. Turn and continue to broil or grill until shrimp and scallops are opaque and slightly brown (about 8 minutes total).
3. If desired, sprinkle with grated lemon zest, more lemon juice and cracked black pepper. Serve.

Per serving
Calories - 148
Total fat - 6 g
Saturated fat - 1 g
Monounsaturated fat - 3 g
Cholesterol - 90 mg
Sodium - 323 mg
Carbohydrate - 2 g
Fiber - 0 g
Protein - 21 g

Exchange list servings
Meat and meat substitutes - 3
Fats - 1

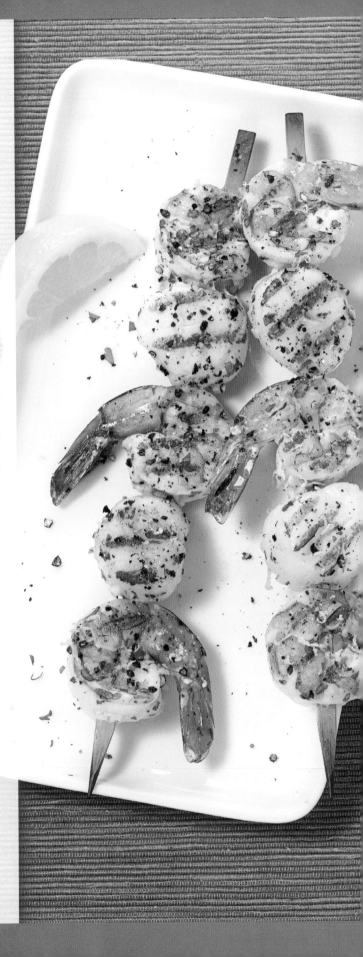

Baby Minted Carrots
Serves 6

Ingredients
6 c. water
1 lb. baby carrots, rinsed
¼ c. apple juice
1 tbsp. cornstarch
½ tbsp. chopped fresh mint leaves
⅛ tsp. ground cinnamon

Preparation
1. Put 6 cups of water into a large saucepan. Add the carrots and boil until tender-crisp, about 10 minutes.
2. Drain the carrots and set aside in a serving bowl.
3. In a separate saucepan over medium heat, combine the apple juice and cornstarch. Stir until the mixture thickens, about 5 minutes. Stir in the mint and cinnamon.
4. Pour the apple juice mixture over the carrots. Serve immediately.

Per serving
Calories - 40
Total fat - 0 g
Saturated fat - 0 g
Monounsaturated fat - 0 g
Cholesterol - 0 mg
Sodium - 45 mg
Carbohydrate - 9 g
Fiber - 2 g
Protein - 1 g

Exchange list servings
Nonstarchy vegetables - 2

Teriyaki Glazed Asparagus
Serves 6

Ingredients
1½ lbs. fresh asparagus, woody ends removed, cut into 1½-inch pieces
2 tbsp. water
½ tsp. sugar
2 tsp. teriyaki sauce

Preparation
1. Place skillet over high heat, add asparagus and water, and cover tightly. Reduce heat to medium. Gently shake skillet to ensure that the asparagus is mixed and evenly heated. Add water as needed so asparagus doesn't burn. This will take about 5 minutes.
2. When asparagus is tender, yet crisp, remove cover and continue to cook until water is almost gone. Remove pan from heat.
3. Sprinkle sugar over asparagus. Drizzle with teriyaki sauce. Gently shake the pan to ensure asparagus is coated evenly with the teriyaki sauce. Serve.

Per serving
Calories - 27
Total fat - 0 g
Saturated fat - 0 g
Monounsaturated fat - 0 g
Cholesterol - 0 mg
Sodium - 115 mg
Carbohydrate - 5 g
Fiber - 2 g
Protein - 3 g

Exchange list servings
Nonstarchy vegetables - 1

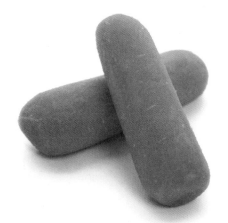

Morning Glory Muffins
Makes 18 small muffins

Ingredients

1 c. all-purpose (plain) flour
1 c. whole-wheat flour
¾ c. sugar
2 tsp. baking soda
2 tsp. ground cinnamon
¼ tsp. salt
¾ c. egg substitute
½ c. vegetable oil
½ c. unsweetened applesauce
2 tsp. vanilla extract
2 c. chopped apples (unpeeled)
½ c. raisins
¾ c. grated carrots
2 tbsp. chopped pecans

Preparation

1. Preheat oven to 350 F.
2. Line a muffin pan with paper or foil liners.
3. In a large bowl, combine the flours, sugar, baking soda, cinnamon and salt. Whisk to blend evenly.
4. In a separate bowl, add the egg substitute, oil, applesauce and vanilla. Stir in the apples, raisins and carrots. Add to the flour mixture and blend just until moistened but still slightly lumpy.
5. Spoon the batter into muffin cups, filling each cup about ⅔ full. Sprinkle with chopped pecans and bake until springy to the touch, about 35 minutes.
6. Let cool for 5 minutes, then transfer the muffins to a wire rack and let cool completely. Serve.

Per serving (1 muffin)

Calories - 175
Total fat - 7 g
Saturated fat - 0.5 g
Monounsaturated fat - 4 g
Cholesterol - 0 mg
Sodium - 195 mg
Carbohydrate - 25 g
Fiber - 2 g
Protein - 3 g

Exchange list servings

Starches - 1
Fruits - ½
Fats - 1

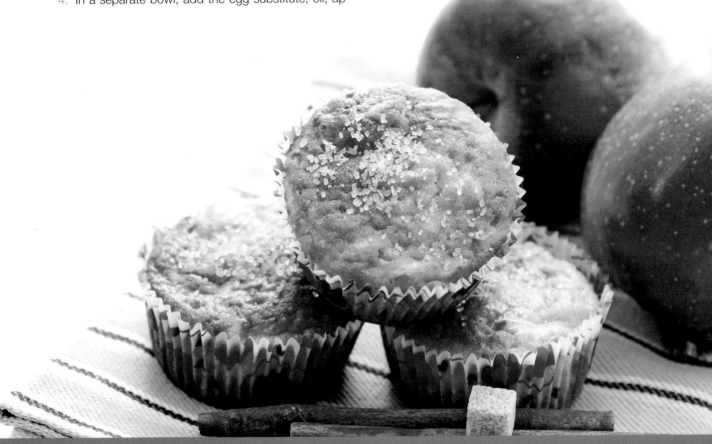

Beef Stew

Serves 8

Ingredients

3 tbsp. whole-wheat flour

1 lb. boneless lean beef stew meat, trimmed of all visible fat and cut into 1½-inch cubes

2 tbsp. olive oil

3 large shallots, thinly sliced

½ tsp. salt (optional)

¾ tsp. black pepper (divided)

½ tsp. dried thyme (or 3 fresh sprigs)

1 bay leaf

3 c. beef or vegetable stock — reduced in sodium, or no salt added

½ c. red wine

6 carrots, cut into 1-inch chunks

6 medium red potatoes, cut into 1-inch chunks

18 small boiling onions, halved (or 1 c. chopped onion)

3 large portobello mushrooms, brushed clean and cut into 1-inch chunks

1 c. celery, cut into 1-inch chunks

⅓ c. parsley, chopped

Preparation

1. Place flour onto plate. Dredge meat in flour. In a large saucepan, heat the oil, add the beef and cook until browned on all sides — about 5 minutes. Remove beef from the pan with a slotted spoon and set aside.

2. Add shallots to the pan and sauté until soft and golden. Add salt, half the pepper, the thyme and bay leaf. Sauté for 1 minute. Return beef to the pan and add the stock and wine. Bring to a boil then reduce heat to low. Cover and simmer until meat is tender — about 40 minutes.

3. Add the carrots, potatoes, onions, mushrooms and celery. Cover and simmer gently until vegetables are tender — about 30 minutes. Stir in the parsley and the remaining pepper.

4. Remove the bay leaf and serve.

Per serving

Calories - 271

Total fat - 7 g

Saturated fat - 2 g

Monounsaturated fat - 4 g

Cholesterol - 32 mg

Sodium - 141 mg

Carbohydrate - 35 g

Fiber - 5 g

Protein - 17 g

Exchange list servings

Starches - 1

Nonstarchy vegetables - 4

Meat and meat substitutes - 2

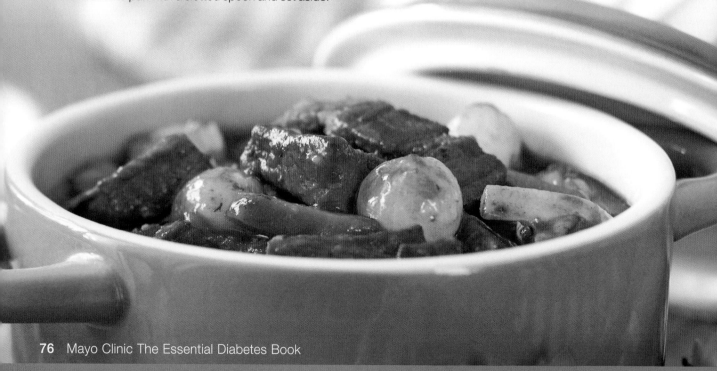

Strawberry Shortcake
Serves 6

Ingredients
1¾ c. all-purpose (plain) flour, sifted
2½ tsp. double-acting baking powder
½ tsp. salt
1 tbsp. sugar
2 tbsp. trans-free margarine
¾ c. fat-free milk
6 c. fresh strawberries, hulled and sliced
¾ c. (6 oz.) fat-free plain yogurt

Preparation
1. Preheat oven to 450 F.
2. Lightly coat a baking sheet with cooking spray.
3. In a large mixing bowl, add the flour, baking powder, salt and sugar. Using a fork, cut the margarine into the dry ingredients until the mixture resembles coarse crumbs. Add the milk and stir just until a moist dough forms.
4. Turn the dough onto a generously floured work surface and, with floured hands, knead gently 6 to 8 times until the dough is smooth and manageable. Using a rolling pin, roll the dough into a rectangle ¼-inch thick. Cut into 6 squares.
5. Place the squares onto the prepared baking sheet. Bake until golden, 10 to 12 minutes.
6. Transfer the biscuits onto individual plates. Top each with 1 cup strawberries and 2 tablespoons yogurt. Serve immediately.

Per serving
Calories - 253
Total fat - 5 g
Saturated fat - 1 g
Monounsaturated fat - 1 g
Cholesterol - 2 mg
Sodium - 481 mg
Carbohydrate - 45 g
Fiber - 4 g
Protein - 7 g

Exchange list servings
Starches - 2
Fruits - 1
Fats - 1

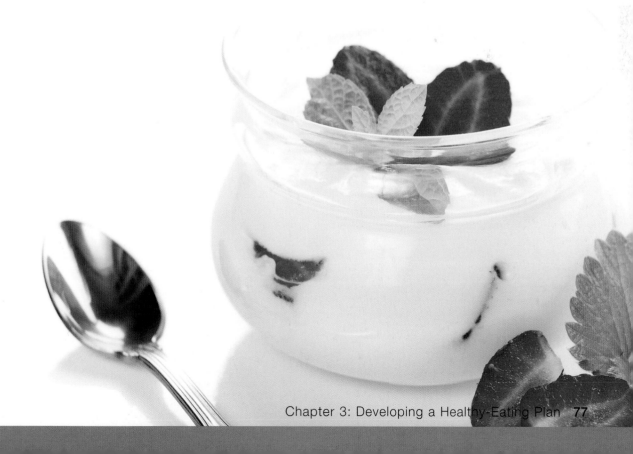

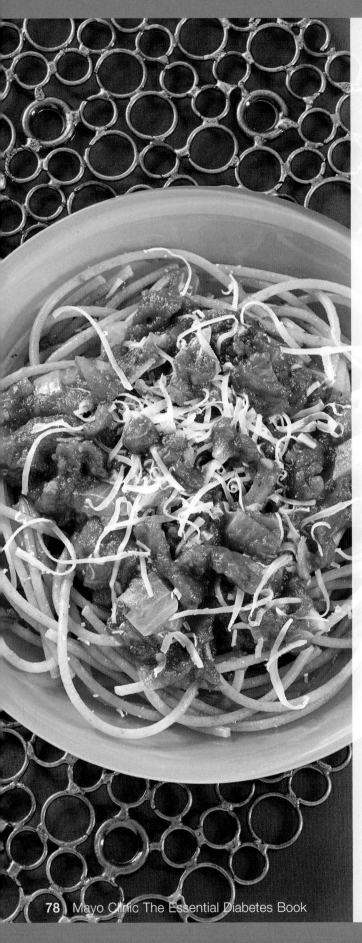

Simple Spaghetti With Marinara Sauce

Serves 8

Ingredients

1 large onion, chopped (1 c.)
2 garlic cloves, minced (or more according to preference)
1 tbsp. olive oil
2 28-oz. cans of whole peeled tomatoes and juice — with no salt added
¼ c. chopped parsley
12 oz. uncooked whole-wheat spaghetti
2 oz. finely grated Parmesan cheese (about ¾ c.)

Preparation

1. In a large skillet, cook onions and garlic in olive oil over medium heat until soft. Add tomatoes including juice and parsley. Simmer, breaking up tomatoes into smaller pieces. (To make thicker sauce, simmer for up to 1½ hours.)
2. Fill a large pot ¾ full with water. Bring to a boil. Add the spaghetti and cook until al dente or until tender, yet with texture. (See package directions for time.) Drain pasta thoroughly.
3. In a large heated bowl, combine the spaghetti and sauce. Toss gently to mix. Serve — each topped with Parmesan cheese.

Per serving

Calories - 257
Total fat - 5 g
Saturated fat - 1.5 g
Monounsaturated fat - 2 g
Cholesterol - 5 mg
Sodium - 143 mg
Carbohydrate - 43 g
Fiber - 7 g
Protein - 10 g

Exchange list servings

Starches - 2
Nonstarchy vegetables - 2
Fats - 1

Heart-Healthy Oatmeal
Serves 6

Ingredients
3¼ c. water
2 c. old-fashioned rolled oats
1 c. blueberries
¼ c. dried cranberries or raisins
¼ c. brown sugar
2 c. fat-free vanilla yogurt, sweetened with low-calorie sweetener
¼ c. chopped walnuts

Preparation
1. In a medium saucepan, bring water to a boil; stir in oats. Return to boil and reduce heat to medium. Cook for about 5 minutes or until most of the liquid is absorbed. Stir frequently.
2. Mix fruit into oatmeal. Spoon into bowls. Top with brown sugar, yogurt and walnuts. Serve.

Per serving
Calories - 258
Total fat - 6 g
Saturated fat - 1 g
Monounsaturated fat - 2 g
Cholesterol - 2 mg
Sodium - 52 mg
Carbohydrate - 42 g
Fiber - 4 g
Protein - 9 g

Exchange list servings
Starches - 1
Fruits - 1
Milk and milk products - ½
Sweets and other carbohydrates - ½
Fats - 1

Breakfast Burrito
Serves 1

Ingredients
½ c. chopped tomato
2 tbsp. chopped onion
¼ c. canned corn, with no added salt
¼ c. egg substitute
1 whole-wheat flour tortilla (6-inch diameter)
2 tbsp. salsa

Preparation
1. In a small skillet, add the chopped tomato, onion and corn. Cook over medium heat until the vegetables are soft and moisture is evaporated.
2. Add the egg substitute and scramble with the vegetables until cooked through, about 3 minutes.
3. To serve, spread the egg mixture in the center of the tortilla and top with salsa. Fold in both sides of the tortilla up over the filling, then roll to close. Serve immediately.

Per serving
Calories - 256
Total fat - 4 g
Saturated fat - 0.5 g
Monounsaturated fat - 1 g
Cholesterol - 1 mg
Sodium - 629 mg
Carbohydrate - 40 g
Fiber - 11 g
Protein - 15 g

Exchange list servings
Starches - 2
Nonstarchy vegetables - 2
Meat and meat substitutes - 1

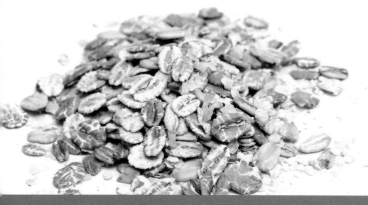

Chicken Pita Sandwich With Lemon Dill Sauce

Serves 8

Ingredients

2 lbs. boneless, skinless chicken breasts, cut into small pieces
2 tsp. olive oil
½ tsp. lemon pepper (unsalted)
1 tbsp. lemon juice
2 medium onions, thinly sliced
2 c. shredded lettuce
4 tomatoes, thinly sliced
2 c. cucumber, thinly sliced
8 whole-wheat pita bread (4-inch diameter)

Sauce:
2 c. fat-free plain yogurt
2 tsp. dried dill weed, or 1½ tbsp. fresh
2 garlic cloves, minced

Preparation

1. In a skillet over medium heat, sauté chicken pieces in 1 teaspoon olive oil until lightly browned and cooked through. About 5 minutes. Sprinkle with lemon pepper and transfer to a bowl. Add the lemon juice; mix with chicken. Cover and keep warm.
2. In the same skillet, heat remaining teaspoon of olive oil and add sliced onions. Sauté until lightly browned and cooked through. Transfer to separate bowl and cover to keep warm.
3. While chicken and onions are cooling, assemble shredded lettuce, sliced tomatoes and cucumbers.
4. Combine all sauce ingredients in a bowl. Mix well.
5. Assemble sandwiches as follows: Place pita on plate. Top with lettuce, tomato and cucumber slices, chicken and onion. Spoon yogurt sauce over chicken and serve.

Per serving (1 pita)

Calories - 276
Total fat - 4 g
Saturated fat - 0.5 g
Monounsaturated fat - 1.5 g
Cholesterol - 67 mg
Sodium - 275 mg
Carbohydrate - 26 g
Fiber - 4 g
Protein - 34 g

Exchange list servings

Starches - 1
Nonstarchy vegetables - 2
Meat and meat substitutes - 3

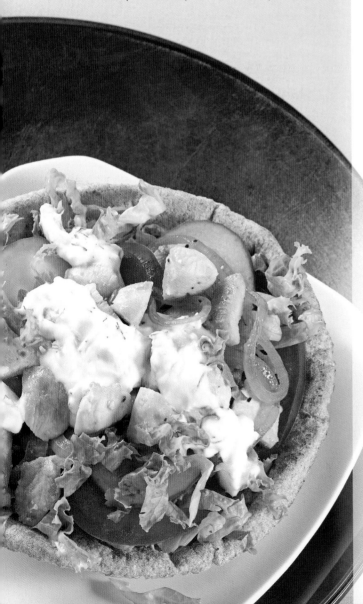

Grilled Salmon With Sliced Cucumber and Radish

Serves 8

Ingredients

2 lbs. salmon fillet
1 tsp. lemon juice
1 tsp. olive oil
Black pepper (optional)
2 c. cucumber, seeded and thinly sliced
¾ c. thinly sliced radishes
1 tsp. olive oil
2 tbsp. vinegar
¼ tsp. dill weed

Preparation

1. Rub salmon with lemon juice, then oil. Sprinkle with black pepper. Cut into 8 pieces. Place salmon, skin-side down, onto aluminum foil that's been sprayed with cooking spray.
2. In a bowl combine the remaining ingredients. Mix well and refrigerate.
3. Grill or broil at medium to high heat until salmon is flaky but still moist. (For best results use a food thermometer — the internal temperature should reach 145 F.)
4. Top each serving of fish with the cucumber and radish mixture.

Per serving

Calories - 168
Total fat - 8 g
Saturated fat - 1 g
Monounsaturated fat - 3 g
Cholesterol - 62 mg
Sodium - 55 mg
Carbohydrate - 1 g
Fiber - trace
Protein - 23 g

Exchange list servings

Free food - 1
Meat and meat substitutes - 3

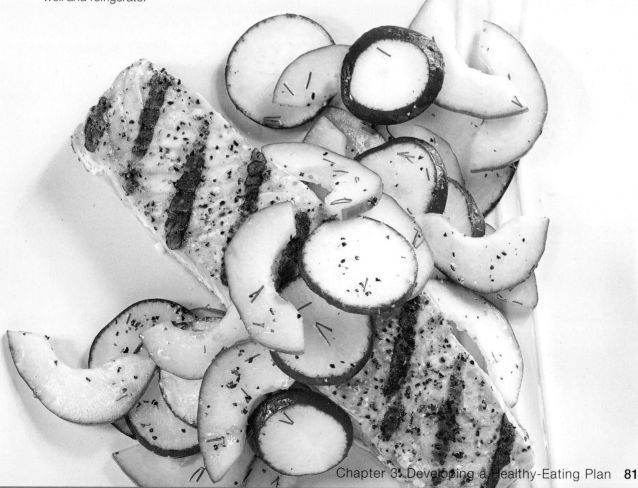

Tropical Fruit Salad
Serves 8

Ingredients
1 mango (about 1½ c. diced)
1 papaya (about 2 c. diced)
2 c. pineapple (fresh, or canned in juice, drained)
4 scallions (including some of the green tops)
1 jalapeno pepper (or 1 tsp. canned green chili pepper)
2 tbsp. lemon or lime juice
2 tbsp. chopped cilantro or parsley

Preparation
1. Dice mango, papaya and pineapple into small uniform pieces. Place into bowl.
2. Chop scallions including some of the green tops into small pieces, add to the fruit.
3. Wearing gloves, remove seeds and white membranes from jalapeno pepper. Chop finely. Add to fruit.
4. Stir in lemon or lime juice and cilantro or parsley. Mix well and serve on a lettuce leaf (as a salad) or as a salsa side dish for fish, seafood or baked chips.

Per serving
Calories - 60
Total fat - trace
Saturated fat - trace
Monounsaturated fat - trace
Cholesterol - 0 mg
Sodium - 11 mg
Carbohydrate - 14 g
Fiber - 2 g
Protein - 1 g

Exchange list servings
Fruits - 1

Apple Cranberry Crisp
Serves 8

Ingredients
6 c. sliced apples (3 peeled, 3 unpeeled)
1 c. fresh cranberries (or frozen unsweetened)
2 tbsp. table sugar
¾ c. rolled oats (uncooked)
⅓ c. brown sugar (lightly packed)
2 tbsp. whole-wheat flour
½ tsp. cinnamon
2 tbsp. trans-free buttery spread
½ c. fat-free vanilla, lemon or maple-flavored yogurt, sweetened with low-calorie sweetener

Preparation
5. Preheat oven to 375 F.
1. In a large mixing bowl combine apples, cranberries, and table sugar. Mix well. Place in a 2-quart square baking dish or a 9-inch pie plate.
2. In a small bowl combine oats, brown sugar, flour, cinnamon and buttery spread. Mix with fingers until crumbly. Sprinkle oat mixture evenly over apple mixture.
3. Bake for 30 to 35 minutes or until apples are tender. Serve warm with a dollop of yogurt.

Per serving
Calories - 176
Total fat - 4 g
Saturated fat - 0.5 g
Monounsaturated fat - 2 g
Cholesterol - trace
Sodium - 51 mg
Carbohydrate - 33 g
Fiber - 4 g
Protein - 2 g

Exchange list servings
Starches - 1
Fruits - 1
Fats - 1

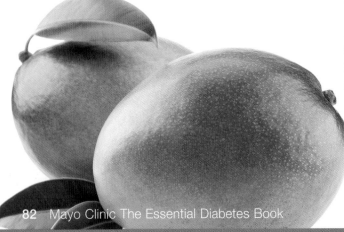

Soft Tacos With Southwestern Vegetables
Serves 4

Ingredients

1 tbsp. olive oil
1 medium red onion, chopped (1 c.)
1 c. diced yellow summer squash
1 c. diced green zucchini
3 large garlic cloves, minced
4 medium tomatoes, seeded and chopped
1 jalapeno pepper, seeded and chopped
1 c. fresh corn kernels (cut from about 2 ears of corn)
or 1 c. frozen corn
1 c. canned pinto or black beans, rinsed and drained
½ c. chopped fresh cilantro
8 corn tortillas
½ c. smoke-flavored salsa

Preparation

1. In a large saucepan, heat the olive oil over medium heat. Add the onion and cook until soft. Add the summer squash and zucchini, and continue cooking until tender, about 5 minutes. Stir in the garlic, tomatoes, jalapeno, corn kernels and beans. Cook until the vegetables are tender-crisp, about 5 minutes. Add the cilantro and remove from the heat.

2. Heat a dry, large frying pan (without a nonstick surface) over medium heat. Add 1 tortilla to the hot pan and heat until softened, about 20 seconds a side. Repeat with the remaining tortillas.

3. To serve, divide the tortillas among individual plates. Spread an equal amount of the vegetable mixture on each tortilla. Top each with 2 tablespoons of the salsa. Serve immediately.

Per serving (2 tacos)

Calories - 310
Total fat - 6 g
Saturated fat - 1 g
Monounsaturated fat - 3 g
Cholesterol - 0 mg
Sodium - 170 mg
Carbohydrate - 54 g
Fiber - 11 g
Protein - 10 g

Exchange list servings

Starches - 3
Nonstarchy vegetables - 2
Fats - 1

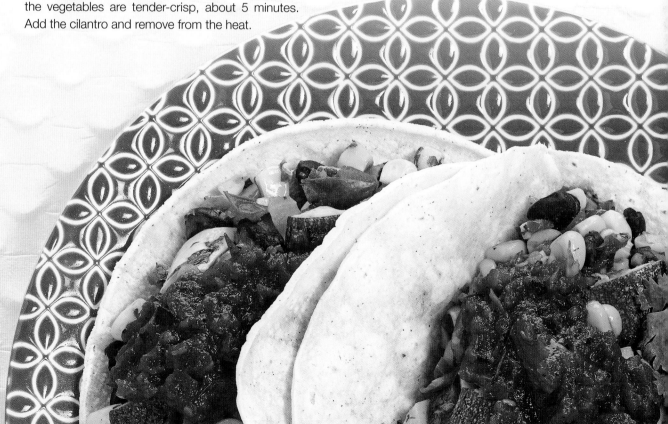

Chapter 4
Achieving a Healthy Weight

Do you need to lose weight? 86

Assess your readiness 88

Set realistic goals 92

Simple first steps 94

The Mayo Clinic Healthy Weight Pyramid 95

Energy density: Eat more and lose weight 98

Keeping a food record 101

What are your eating triggers? 103

What's your meal routine? 104

Adapting recipes 106

Be a smart shopper 107

Bumps in the road: Overcoming setbacks 109

A visit with Dr. Donald Hensrud

"The good news is that weight loss can reverse this process and the effect can be immediate. Within a couple of days of losing weight, blood glucose values improve, sometimes dramatically."

The main risk factors for type 2 diabetes are a family history of diabetes, being overweight (particularly around the abdomen), a sedentary lifestyle and diet. Of these, the most important risk factor you can control is body weight. But keep in mind that physical activity and diet also influence weight. As you well may know, the main reason the prevalence of diabetes is increasing in the United States is that the number of people who are overweight or obese is increasing.

When it comes to diabetes, the hormone insulin is a key factor — it helps lower blood sugar (glucose) by helping transport glucose into cells. The way excess weight increases your risk of diabetes is that as you gain weight, insulin doesn't work as well in your body to lower blood glucose — your body becomes resistant to insulin's effects. Initially, your body produces more insulin to overcome this resistance. But as time goes by, your body becomes even more resistant to insulin and it can't keep increasing production. Finally, blood glucose values start to rise and you develop diabetes.

The good news is that weight loss can reverse this process, and the effect can be immediate. Within a couple of days of losing weight, blood glucose values improve, sometimes dramatically. The best way to lose weight is through lifestyle changes — changing what and how much you eat and being more physically active. In some cases, diabetes can be completely reversed and blood glucose values can return to normal or near normal.

There are other reasons to manage your weight. Diabetes increases your risk of eye disease, kidney disease, nerve damage and particularly heart disease. Positive lifestyle changes that produce weight loss will decrease your risk of these conditions. In addition, weight loss can help improve other health conditions related to being overweight, including high blood pressure, abnormal blood fats (lipids), obstruc-

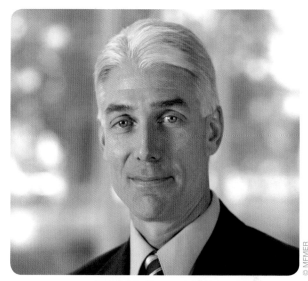

Donald D. Hensrud, M.D.
Preventive Medicine

tive sleep apnea and more. Finally, eating better and getting more exercise will simply help you feel better.

When making changes in your diet, it's important not only to decrease total calories, but also to choose foods that are healthy, taste good and are practical to eat every day. Healthy eating and improving your weight are possible if they're done in the right manner with a positive attitude.

Similarly, exercise doesn't have to be drudgery. Many people say that when they're more active, they feel better. Increasing general physical activity throughout the day is an effective strategy to burn calories. With exercise, it's best to start by doing just a little bit each day, and gradually increase the amount and intensity over time.

Healthy-lifestyle habits can give you the best chance to treat your diabetes and prevent health complications. Yes, losing weight takes work — or more correctly planning — but the rewards are great. With the right attitude, you can have fun and feel great while adding years to your life!

Being overweight is by far the greatest risk factor for type 2 diabetes. An overwhelming majority of people who develop this type of diabetes are overweight. By contrast, most people with type 1 diabetes are at or below their ideal weight.

Why is weight such an important factor in type 2 diabetes? Fat alters how your body's cells respond to the hormone insulin — it causes them to become resistant to insulin's effects, reducing the amount of blood sugar (glucose) that's transported into your cells. As a result, more glucose remains in your bloodstream, increasing your blood glucose level.

The good news is that you can reverse this process. As you lose weight, your cells become more responsive to insulin, allowing the hormone to do its job. For some people with type 2 diabetes, losing weight is all that's necessary to control their diabetes and return their blood glucose to normal.

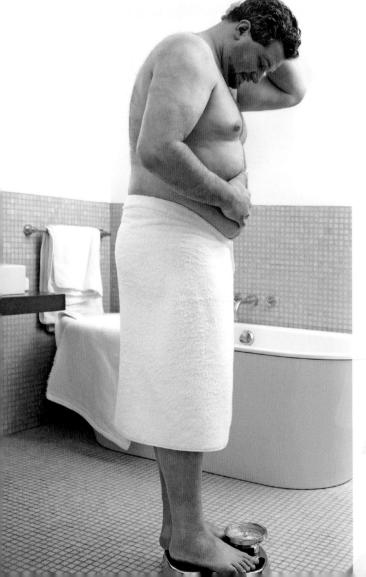

And the amount of weight you need to lose to see benefits doesn't have to be extreme. A modest weight loss of 5 to 10 percent of your weight can lower your blood glucose level, as well as provide many other health benefits, such as reducing your blood pressure and blood cholesterol levels.

Losing weight can be a challenge — as you well may know. However, with a positive attitude and the right advice, it's a challenge you can meet. As you develop healthier habits, the pounds will gradually begin to come off.

Do you need to lose weight?

Before figuring out if you're overweight by medical standards, keep in mind that many fashion models and celebrities are unrealistically thin, and you shouldn't expect to look like them. Your goal is to achieve a healthy weight — one that improves your blood glucose control and reduces your risk of other medical problems.

To see if you could benefit from weight loss, consider these three factors — your body mass index, your waist circumference, and your personal and family medical history.

Body mass index

Body mass index (BMI) is a measurement based on a formula that takes into account your weight and height in determining whether you have a healthy or unhealthy percentage of body fat. To estimate your BMI, use the chart on the next page.

A BMI under 18.5 indicates that you're underweight, 18.5 to 24.9 is considered a healthy range, 25 to 29.9 indicates overweight, and 30 or greater means you're obese.

The BMI is a helpful guide, but it's not perfect. For example, muscle weighs more than fat, and many people who are very muscular and physically fit have high BMIs without added health risks.

What's your BMI?

To determine your body mass index (BMI), find your height in the left column. Follow that row across until you reach the column with the weight nearest yours. Look at the top of the column for your approximate BMI.

	Normal		Overweight					Obese				
BMI	**19**	**24**	**25**	**26**	**27**	**28**	**29**	**30**	**35**	**40**	**45**	**50**
Height					Weight in pounds							
4'10"	91	115	119	124	129	134	138	143	167	191	215	239
4'11"	94	119	124	128	133	138	143	148	173	198	222	247
5'0"	97	123	128	133	138	143	148	153	179	204	230	255
5'1"	100	127	132	137	143	148	153	158	185	211	238	264
5'2"	104	131	136	142	147	153	158	164	191	218	246	273
5'3"	107	135	141	146	152	158	163	169	197	225	254	282
5'4"	110	140	145	151	157	163	169	174	204	232	262	291
5'5"	114	144	150	156	162	168	174	180	210	240	270	300
5'6"	118	148	155	161	167	173	179	186	216	247	278	309
5'7"	121	153	159	166	172	178	185	191	223	255	287	319
5'8"	125	158	164	171	177	184	190	197	230	262	295	328
5'9"	128	162	169	176	182	189	196	203	236	270	304	338
5'10"	132	167	174	181	188	195	202	209	243	278	313	348
5'11"	136	172	179	186	193	200	208	215	250	286	322	358
6'0"	140	177	184	191	199	206	213	221	258	294	331	368
6'1"	144	182	189	197	204	212	219	227	265	302	340	378
6'2"	148	186	194	202	210	218	225	233	272	311	350	389
6'3"	152	192	200	208	216	224	232	240	279	319	359	399
6'4"	156	197	205	213	221	230	238	246	287	328	369	410

National Institutes of Health, 1998
Asians with a BMI of 23 or higher may have an increased risk of health problems

Waist circumference

Another way of determining if you're at a healthy weight is to measure your waist circumference. If you carry most of your weight around your waist or upper body, you have an apple shape. If you carry most of your fat around your hips and thighs, you have a pear shape.

Generally, it's better to have a pear shape than an apple shape. That's because excess fat around your abdomen is linked with greater risk of weight-related diseases such as type 2 diabetes and heart disease.

To determine whether you're carrying too much weight around your abdomen, measure your waist circumference at its smallest point, usually at the level of your navel. If you're a man with a waist more than 40 inches or a woman with a waist more than 35 inches, you're at higher risk of health problems. The greater the waist measurement, the greater the risk.

Personal history

An evaluation of your medical history is equally important in determining if your weight is healthy.

▶ Do you have a health condition that would benefit from weight loss? For most people with type 2 diabetes, the answer to this question is yes. This is especially important if you also have another condition that would benefit from weight loss, such as hypertension.
▶ Have you gained much weight since high school? Weight gain in adulthood is associated with increased health risks.
▶ Do you smoke cigarettes, have more than two alcoholic drinks a day or live with too much stress?

In combination with these behaviors, excess weight has greater health implications.

Your results

If your BMI indicates that you aren't overweight and you're not carrying too much weight around your abdomen, there's probably no health advantage to changing your weight. Your weight is healthy.

If your BMI is 25 to 29.9 and your waist circumference exceeds healthy guidelines, you could probably benefit from losing a few pounds, especially if you answered yes to at least one personal health question above.

Discuss your weight with your doctor during your next checkup. If your BMI is 30 or more, losing weight can improve your overall health and reduce your risk of serious weight-related diseases, including complications of diabetes.

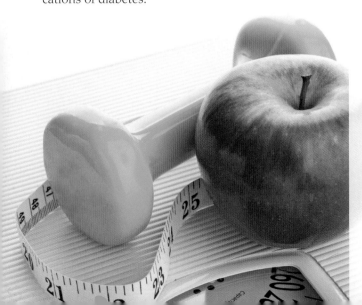

Assess your readiness

You need to decide whether now is the right time to start a weight-loss program. It's OK if it's not. Starting before you're ready can set you up for failure. But you don't want to put off your start date any longer than necessary, especially if your health is at risk. The questions on the next page may help you make your decision.

Why readiness is important

If you're going to lose weight because you want to — and not because you think it's expected of you — you'll quickly appreciate the benefits that come from weight loss. If you feel positive about most of your responses, start your weight-loss program now. The fewer obstacles you have, the more likely you are to establish healthy eating and fitness habits in place of unhealthy habits.

If you're not ready to start

If you're uncertain about many of the questions on the next page, consider waiting for a better time. Whether you decide to start or delay, review the obstacles to losing weight and possible solutions on pages 90 and 91.

If you're not ready to start a weight-loss program, talk with your health care provider and come up with ideas on how to prepare yourself. For example:

▶ If you're under a lot of stress, would you benefit from a stress management course?
▶ If this is an emotional time for you, for whatever reason, where can you get support?
▶ If a hectic schedule is an issue, how can you prioritize, trim your task list and make time for yourself?

Looking ahead

Set a date to reassess your readiness. Even if you're not ready to move ahead full force, consider taking a few simple steps first (see page 94).

Are you ready?

1. How motivated are you to lose weight?
   a. Highly motivated
   b. Moderately motivated
   c. Somewhat motivated
   d. Slightly motivated or not at all

2. Considering the amount of stress affecting your life right now, to what extent can you focus on weight loss and on making lifestyle changes?
   a. Can focus easily
   b. Can focus relatively well
   c. Uncertain
   d. Can focus somewhat or not at all

3. It's best to lose weight at a steady rate of 1 to 2 pounds a week. How realistic are your expectations about how much weight you'd like to lose and how fast you want to lose it?
   a. Very realistic
   b. Moderately realistic
   c. Somewhat realistic
   d. Slightly or very unrealistic

4. Aside from special celebrations, do you ever eat a lot of food rapidly while feeling that your eating is out of control?
   a. No
   b. Yes

5. If you answered yes to the previous question, how often have you eaten like this during the last year?
   a. About once a month or less
   b. A few times a month
   c. About once a week
   d. About three times a week or more

6. Do you eat for emotional reasons, for example, when you feel anxious, depressed, angry or lonely?
   a. Never or rarely
   b. Occasionally
   c. Frequently
   d. Always

7. How confident are you that you can make changes in your eating habits and maintain them?
   a. Completely confident
   b. Moderately confident
   c. Somewhat confident
   d. Slightly confident or not at all

8. How confident are you that you can exercise several times a week?
   a. Completely confident
   b. Moderately confident
   c. Somewhat confident
   d. Slightly confident or not at all

If most of your responses are:

▶ **a and b,** you're probably ready to start a weight-loss program.
▶ **b and c,** consider if you're ready or if you should wait and take action to prepare yourself.
▶ **d,** you may want to hold off on your start date and take steps to prepare yourself. Reassess your readiness again soon.

Note: If your answer to question 5 was b, c or d, discuss this with your doctor. If you have an eating disorder, it's crucial that you get appropriate treatment.

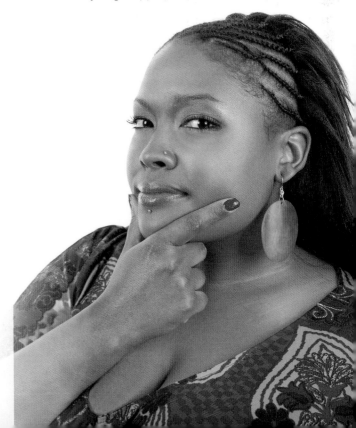

Action guide to weight-loss barriers

To lose weight — and maintain a healthy weight — you need to identify your barriers to weight loss and find solutions. Check all the barriers that apply to you.

Barriers	Possible solutions
❑ I tried to lose weight before, but it didn't work. So I don't have a lot of confidence that it will work this time.	› Set realistic expectations. › Focus on behavioral changes rather than numbers of pounds. › Make small changes to your lifestyle so that you don't give up. › When you have a setback, start fresh the next day. › Write down previous obstacles and strategies for dealing with them. › Identify what will motivate you to be successful.
❑ My family doesn't like to try new foods, and it's too much work to prepare two different meals.	› Take it slow. Make a few small changes each week. › Keep fruit in a location where it's visible and easy to grab. › Prepare a favorite dish using a different cooking method, such as baking chicken instead of frying. › Ask family members which healthy foods they'd like to try. Give them several options so that they might be more willing to experiment.
❑ I don't like vegetables and fruits.	› Find a few that you do like and eat them more often. › Try vegetables that you've never had. Add them to your favorite soups or replace some of the meat in casseroles or pizzas with vegetables. › Include fresh fruit with your cereal, and stir fruit into low-fat yogurt or low-fat cottage cheese.
❑ I can't resist certain foods that I shouldn't eat, such as potato chips and other junk foods.	› Avoid keeping junk food at home. › If you can't resist the urge, buy only a small amount, such as a single serving. Have it along with your meal. › Eat healthy foods first, so you won't be so hungry when you eat your favorites. › Try healthier versions, such as baked rather than regular chips.
❑ I eat when I'm stressed, depressed or bored.	› Instead of high-fat, high-calorie comfort foods, keep healthy foods in your house. › Try to distract yourself from eating by calling a friend, running an errand or going for a walk. Try to think positively. For example, write down what you want to achieve with weight loss.

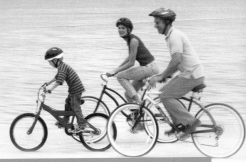

Barriers	Possible solutions
❏ I don't have time to make healthy meals.	❯ Keep it simple. For example, serve a fresh salad with fat-free dressing, a whole-grain roll and a piece of fruit. ❯ Stop at a deli or grocery store and buy a healthy sandwich, soup or entree that's low in calories and fat.
❏ When eating out, I like to eat my favorite foods — not something healthy.	❯ Eat only half of your favorite foods and save the other half for the next day. (But if you dine out often, make healthy eating a routine.) ❯ If you know that you'll be eating extra calories, increase your exercise for the day.
❏ I don't like to exercise.	❯ Remember that physical activity — anything that gets you moving — burns calories, too. ❯ Choose activities that you enjoy and include variety. ❯ Exercise with a friend or a group so that you can socialize. ❯ Take a class or buy an exercise DVD if you need structure.
❏ I'm too tired to exercise.	❯ Regular physical activity increases energy. Begin with just 10 minutes of activity — a little is better than none. ❯ Exercise when your energy is highest, whether it's in the morning, afternoon or early evening. Keep motivational messages where you'll see them often.
❏ I was slowly losing weight, but now I'm not anymore, and I haven't changed my diet.	❯ You may have reached a plateau. Consider reducing your calorie intake by 200 calories, unless this puts you too low. ❯ Gradually increase your exercise time by 15 to 30 minutes. If possible, also increase the intensity. Get more physically active throughout the day, such as taking the stairs instead of the elevator at work.
❏ Other barriers	❯ Other solutions

Set realistic goals

Goal setting puts your thoughts into action. But your ability to reach weight goals is closely tied to how realistic your expectations are. Goals that are unrealistic or too long term just set you up for frustration and disappointment.

Include both process goals and outcome goals.

▶ A process goal measures specific activities. For example, rather than vowing to lose 20 pounds, commit to walking for 30 minutes a day, five days a week.

▶ An outcome goal is generally longer term and measures the end result but not how you achieve the result — for example, a goal to lose 20 pounds.

Be SMART about your goals

Set goals that are SMART: specific, measurable, attainable, relevant and time-limited.

Specific

State exactly what you want to achieve, how you're going to do it and when you want to achieve it.

Measurable

Track your progress. For example, if your goal is to eat more servings of vegetables and fruits, track the number of servings you eat each day in a food record or food diary. If your goal is to walk for 30 minutes a day or jog 3 miles a day five days a week, track this in an exercise log. Review your progress each week.

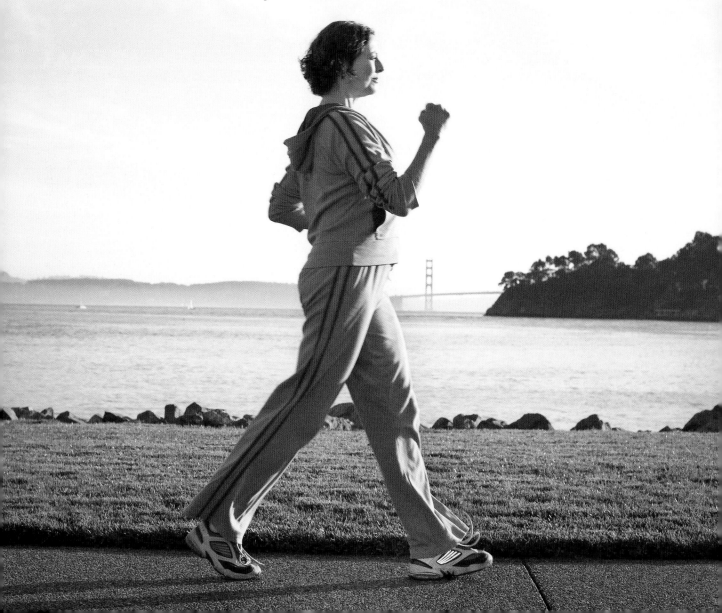

Attainable

Ask yourself whether a goal is reasonable before you set it. Tailor your expectations to your personal situation. Are you allowing enough time and resources? Start slowly and work your way up to larger goals.

Relevant

Pick a goal that's relevant for you at the stage you're at in life. Think about what's most important to you and what will truly benefit your life.

Time-limited

It's helpful to plan a series of small goals that build on each other instead of one major long-term goal. Setting and achieving short-term goals helps keep you motivated. Choose a definite start date.

....

Remember: Make a commitment and don't look too far ahead. What can you do today to make this weight-loss plan work for you?

Write down your goals

Work with a weight-loss or diabetes educator to develop your process and outcome goals. Talk about what worked and what didn't work well in the past and why. Were your goals SMART? What can you do differently this time around to increase your chance of success?

Write down your initial goals and review them often. But remember that your goals may change over time. If so, add your new ones.

Reassess and adjust your goals or your plan

When you struggle with your weight program, be willing to reassess and adjust your goals — or your plan to achieve them. You may need to change your goals so that they're a better fit for your needs. Talk with a weight-loss or diabetes educator. Make sure all of the goals are yours and not someone else's. Keep them realistic.

Remember, you will lose weight. And your life will change. But it takes time and commitment.

You have the power!

Don't sell yourself — and your efforts — short.

Recognize your success. When you do well and meet your goals, congratulate yourself on your effort and self-control. Don't give your weight program the credit. You did it. The program just guided you.

Reward yourself. Celebrate reaching short-term as well as long-term goals. Consider what you've already accomplished — whether it's changing your diet, getting more physically active, going down one size in clothing, or walking a flight of stairs without getting winded. Reward yourself with a fun day trip or a new CD, or simply take time to relax.

Cheer yourself on. If you get discouraged about continuing on, write down why you feel better as a result of your weight loss up to this point. Look at how you've succeeded in changing your eating and activity habits. You may reap benefits that you never anticipated.

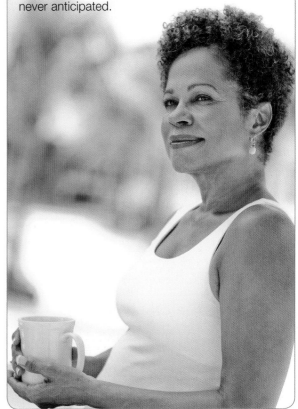

Simple first steps

You're eager to start losing weight. But you don't have time to read the details about another new approach. Or you're overwhelmed by the thought of another new approach, and you just want some simple first steps. What can you do now?

Choose one or more of the steps outlined in the table below to get started toward developing a healthier you. While simple, they are significant measures you can take to begin dropping pounds.

After two weeks, if you're ready, move on to the full program that begins on page 95 — and start reaping the benefits.

What I'll do	How I'll do it
I'll eat more fruit each day instead of sweets.	▶ I'll put out a bowl of fruit at home so that it's easy to grab. ▶ I'll eat low-fat fruit yogurt. ▶ I'll eat fruit at the beginning or end of meals.
I'll eat more vegetables each day, and I'll eat less meat.	▶ I'll buy ready-to-eat, snack-size veggies, such as cherry tomatoes or baby carrots. ▶ I'll eat a salad with a variety of colorful veggies at lunch or supper. ▶ I'll put more veggies and less meat on my plate.
I'll increase my physical activity on most days of the week.	▶ I'll take the stairs instead of the elevator. ▶ I'll park farther away from my destination. ▶ I'll ride my bike instead of driving my car. ▶ I'll walk first thing in the morning or as soon as I get home. ▶ I'll walk at lunchtime with a co-worker.

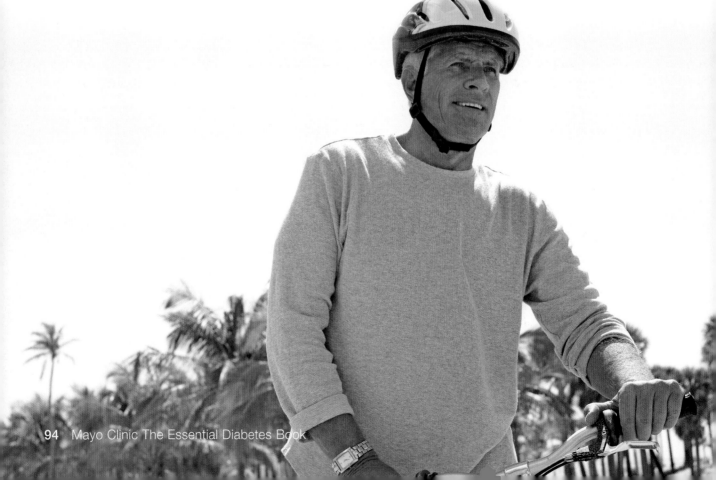

The Mayo Clinic Healthy Weight Pyramid

The same healthy-eating plan for controlling your blood glucose can also help you lose weight, as long as you pay attention to the total amount of calories you consume each day. For many people, simply replacing a few servings of fats, dairy products or meat with lower calorie vegetables, fruits and whole grains is enough to reach their calorie goal.

Small changes also add up. For example, by switching from whole milk to fat-free milk, you save 60 calories a cup. If you drink a cup of milk each day, that's 420 calories a week. Over time, simple steps can save a lot of calories.

Mayo Clinic has developed a common-sense approach to weight control that encourages smart decisions and healthy behaviors grounded on the fundamentals of the Mayo Clinic Healthy Weight Pyramid. Instead of a diet that you go on and off, it's a lifestyle program to better your health.

The Mayo Clinic approach recognizes that successful, long-term weight loss needs to focus on more than just the food you eat and the pounds you lose. It needs to focus on your overall health and well-being.

A key element of the Mayo Clinic Healthy Weight Pyramid — shown in the center of the pyramid below — is incorporating physical activity into your daily routine. You'll read more about physical activity in the next chapter.

A note about the recommended number of daily servings: When a range is shown, the lower number of servings is based on 1,200 daily calories and the higher number is based on 2,000 daily calories.

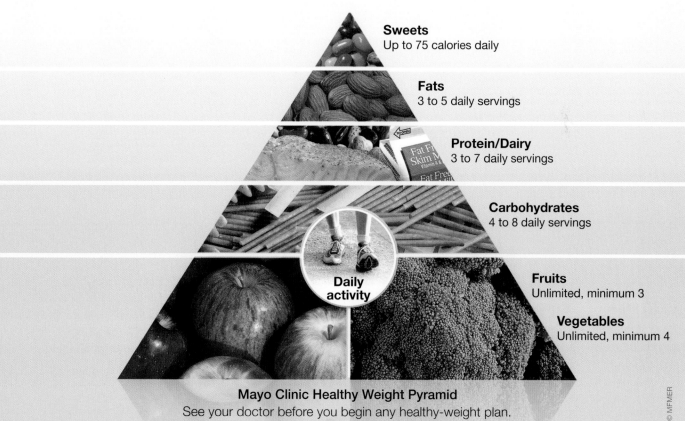

Sweets
Up to 75 calories daily

Fats
3 to 5 daily servings

Protein/Dairy
3 to 7 daily servings

Carbohydrates
4 to 8 daily servings

Daily activity

Fruits
Unlimited, minimum 3

Vegetables
Unlimited, minimum 4

Mayo Clinic Healthy Weight Pyramid
See your doctor before you begin any healthy-weight plan.

© MFMER

Food groups: Your best food choices

Here's a look at the food groups that make up the Mayo Clinic Healthy Weight Pyramid. Keep in mind that serving sizes are important.

Vegetables

A nutritional powerhouse, most vegetables are low in calories and fat and high in fiber. Focus on fresh vegetables, but frozen or canned without added fat or salt are OK. Go for variety. *Note:* Starchy, higher calorie vegetables (such as corn, potatoes and winter squash) are counted as carbohydrates.

Fruits

Practically all types of fruit fit into a healthy diet. But whole fresh, frozen and canned fruits without added sugar are better choices. They're filling and packed with nutrients and fiber. Different colors have different nutrients, so eat a variety. Limit fruit juices and dried fruits — they have more calories and are less filling than whole fruits.

Carbohydrates

Most foods in this group are grains or made from grains. Whole grains are best because they're higher in fiber and other important nutrients. Examples include whole-grain cereal, whole-wheat bread, whole-wheat pasta and oatmeal. Look for the term *whole* as one of the first ingredients on the label.

Daily calorie goal for healthy weight loss

To lose weight, the following daily calorie goals often work well.

Weight	Starting calorie goal	
Pounds	Women	Men
250 or less	1,200	1,400
251 to 300	1,400	1,600
301 or more	1,600	1,800

Protein and dairy

The best protein and dairy choices are those that are high in protein but low in saturated fat and calories, such as legumes — beans, peas and lentils, which are also good sources of fiber — fish, skinless white meat poultry, fat-free dairy products and egg whites.

Fats

Your body needs certain types of fat to function properly, but saturated fats and trans fats increase your risk of heart disease. Focus on good fats (see page 55).

Sweets

This group includes candies, cakes, cookies, pies, doughnuts and other desserts, as well as table sugar. Most of these foods are high in calories and fat without any nutrients. With sweets, keep this phrase in mind — small is beautiful.

Tailor the pyramid to meet your needs

Use the Mayo Clinic Healthy Weight Pyramid in a way that works best for your needs. Here's how to get started:

▶ **Determine your calorie goal.** To lose weight, follow the daily calorie goals shown at left, unless your doctor advises otherwise. If you feel exceptionally hungry at this calorie level — despite eating lots of vegetables and fruits — or you're losing weight faster than desired, move up to the next calorie level.

Fewer than 1,200 calories a day for women and 1,400 calories a day for men generally isn't recommended — you may not get enough nutrients. But don't become so focused on calories that you lose sight of the big picture — adopting a healthier lifestyle.

▶ **Determine the number of servings.** Use the table on the next page to determine the number of servings to eat each day. Eat as many fresh or frozen vegetables and fruits as you like — they're low in calories and packed with nutrition. Adjust your goals as necessary. If, for example, you don't reach your vegetable goal on Monday, eat extra vegetables on Tuesday.

Daily serving recommendations for different calorie levels

Food group	Starting calorie goal				
	1,200	1,400	1,600	1,800	2,000
Vegetables*	4 or more	4 or more	5 or more	5 or more	5 or more
Fruits*	3 or more	4 or more	5 or more	5 or more	5 or more
	4	5	6	7	8
Protein/dairy†	3	4	5	6	7
Fats†	3	3	3	4	5
Sweets†	75 calories a day				

*The servings for fruits and vegetables are minimums — eat as much as you like.
†The recommended servings for carbohydrates, protein/dairy, fats and sweets are maximums.

▸ **Learn serving sizes.** Many people regularly eat more than they should because they don't know how to estimate a serving size. Use the visual cues on page 59 to help you gauge what equates to a serving.

▸ **Keep a daily food record.** This has helped many people to successfully lose unwanted pounds. Throughout the day, record what foods you eat, the amount, the number of servings of each and the food groups to which they belong. Or track this data using your computer or phone. Too much information? Write a short summary each day. Consider writing your thoughts and feelings in a food journal.

▸ **Include physical activity in your day.** Whether it's informal, such as brisk walking, or structured exercise, move as much as you can during the day. The key to keeping physically active is making it convenient.

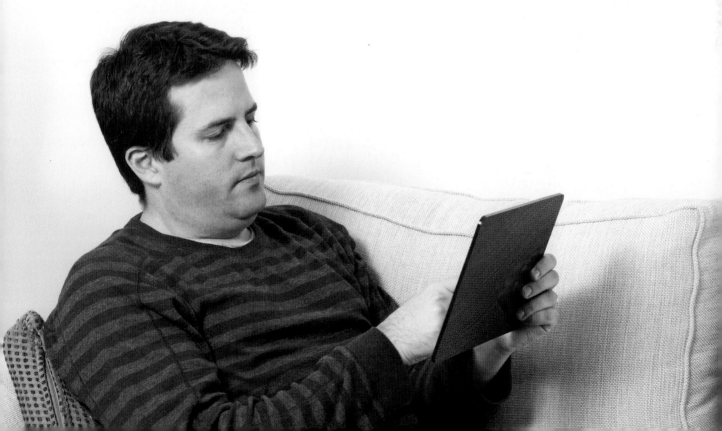

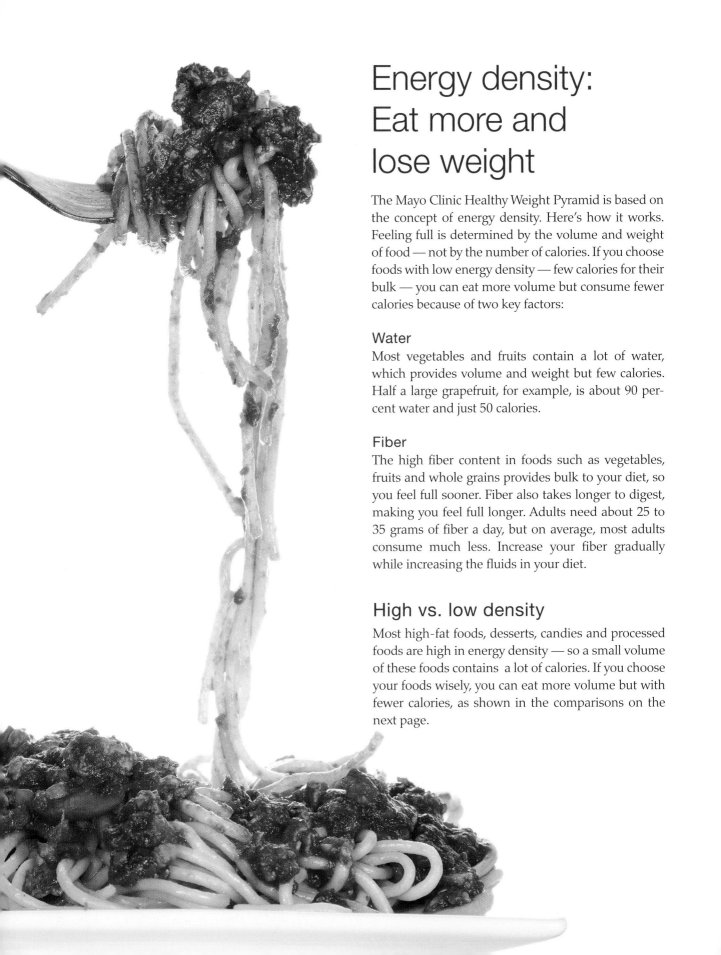

Energy density: Eat more and lose weight

The Mayo Clinic Healthy Weight Pyramid is based on the concept of energy density. Here's how it works. Feeling full is determined by the volume and weight of food — not by the number of calories. If you choose foods with low energy density — few calories for their bulk — you can eat more volume but consume fewer calories because of two key factors:

Water

Most vegetables and fruits contain a lot of water, which provides volume and weight but few calories. Half a large grapefruit, for example, is about 90 percent water and just 50 calories.

Fiber

The high fiber content in foods such as vegetables, fruits and whole grains provides bulk to your diet, so you feel full sooner. Fiber also takes longer to digest, making you feel full longer. Adults need about 25 to 35 grams of fiber a day, but on average, most adults consume much less. Increase your fiber gradually while increasing the fluids in your diet.

High vs. low density

Most high-fat foods, desserts, candies and processed foods are high in energy density — so a small volume of these foods contains a lot of calories. If you choose your foods wisely, you can eat more volume but with fewer calories, as shown in the comparisons on the next page.

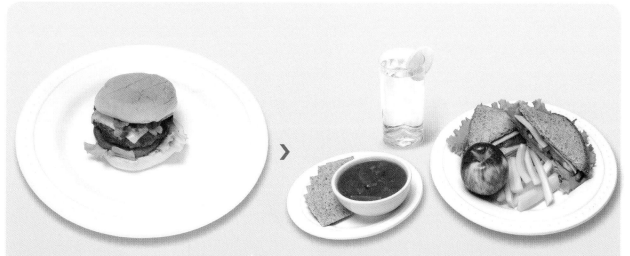

High-energy-dense lunch — 595 calories
Bacon cheeseburger (thick patty)

Low-energy-dense lunch — 556 calories
Roast turkey breast (3 ounces) sandwich on whole-wheat bread with low-fat cheese (1 ounce), lettuce and tomatoes, plus an apple, celery sticks, vegetable soup (1 cup), whole-grain crackers and water with lemon slice

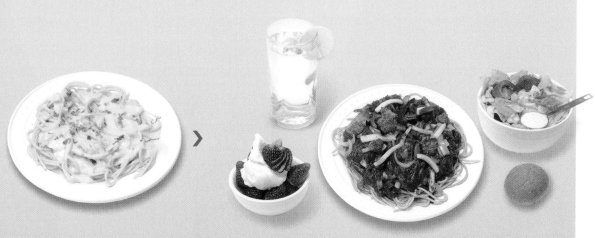

High-energy-dense supper — 646 calories
Spaghetti (¾ cup) with cheese sauce (¾ cup)

Low-energy-dense supper — 622 calories
Whole-wheat spaghetti (1 cup) and fat-free spaghetti sauce (1 cup) topped with broccoli, sweet bell peppers, onions and zucchini, plus whole-grain roll, side salad (with 1 tablespoon fat-free dressing), strawberries (1½ cups) topped with fat-free frozen vanilla yogurt (½ cup) and water with lemon slice

What about all those fad diets?

In general, fad diets can be risky to your health. And most people stick with fad diets for only a short while before they go off them and eventually gain their weight back. If a diet sounds too good to be true, it probably is. The reason why there are so many fad diets is that none of them has led to lasting weight loss and improved health.

Whether a diet is low carb, low fat or somewhere in between, here are a few points to keep in mind:

▶ Calories count. To lose weight, the number of calories you consume needs to be less than the calories you expend.

▶ To keep weight off, your diet needs to be practical, enjoyable and suitable to your lifestyle.

▶ Both low-carb and low-fat diets can be made healthier with good food choices, such as emphasized in the Mayo Clinic Healthy Weight Pyramid.

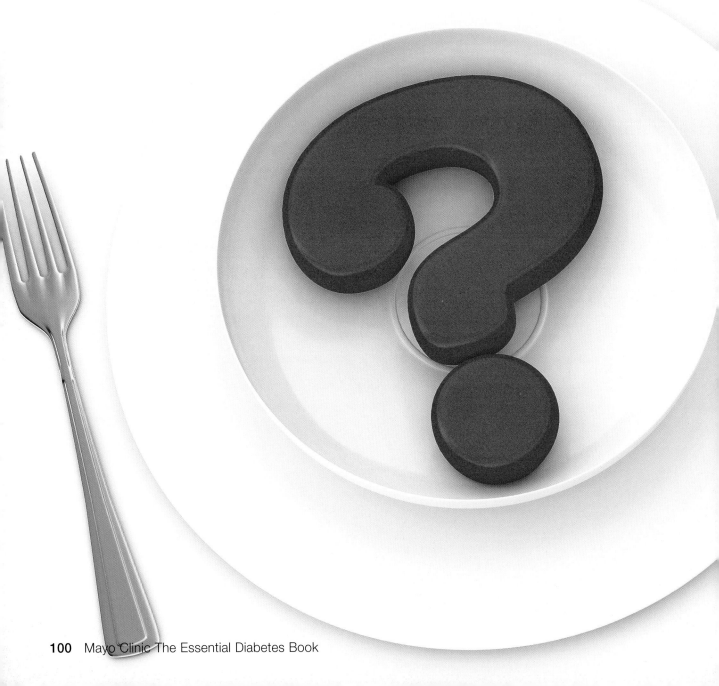

Keeping a food record

Most people underestimate the amount of food they eat by at least 20 percent. Research shows that people who record what they eat each day are often more successful at losing weight. When you first begin your weight-loss program, a daily food record can help you see how much you actually eat in a day and where you need to make improvements.

	Food*	Amount	Servings	Food groups
Breakfast	Whole-wheat flake cereal, dry	1 cup	2	Carbohydrates
	Skim milk	1 cup	1	Protein/dairy
	Banana	1 small	1	Fruits
Snack	Orange	1 medium	1	Fruits
Lunch	Greek salad			
	Spinach	2 cups	1	Vegetables
	Tomato, medium	1	1	Vegetables
	Green pepper, cucumber	½ each	1	Vegetables
	Olive oil	2 teaspoons	2	Fats
	Bread, whole-grain	1 slice	1	Carbohydrates
Snack	Apple	1 small	1	Fruits
Supper	Fish (cod, salmon, tuna)	3 ounces	1	Protein/dairy
	Pasta (whole-grain)	½ cup	1	Carbohydrates
	Tomato sauce	¼ cup	1	Vegetables
	Salad			
	Lettuce	2 cups	1	Vegetables
	Cherry tomatoes	8 tomatoes	1	Vegetables
	Fat-free French dressing	2 tablespoons	1	Fats
Snack	Strawberries	1½ cups	1	Fruits

*Calorie-free beverages, such as black coffee, unsweetened iced tea or sparkling water, don't count.

Beverages: How many calories are you drinking?

Although some beverages, such as juice and milk, have important nutrients, they also contain a lot of calories. Drinking reduced-calorie ("light") juices or diluting juices with plain or sparkling water can help lower calories. But whole fruit, packed with fiber and nutrients, is a much better choice and more filling. To help cut calories in milk yet still get your calcium, switch to low-fat or fat-free milk. Water is still the best choice when it comes to satisfying thirst and cutting the urge to snack. Try sparkling water if you don't like plain water.

Calories in common beverages

Beverage	Serving size*	Average calories[†]
Water	8 oz.	0
Coffee	8 oz.	2
Tea, hot or cold, brewed with water (unsweetened)	8 oz.	0-2
Tea, iced (presweetened with sugar), ready to drink	20 oz.	150-240
Milk, whole	8 oz.	150-160
Milk, 2%	8 oz.	120-140
Milk, 1%	8 oz.	100-120
Milk, fat-free	8 oz.	90-100
Fruit juice (100%, no added sugar), ready to drink	8 oz.	100-180
Fruit drinks	8 oz.	100-150
Soda, regular	20 oz.	205-315
Soda, diet (artificially sweetened)	20 oz.	0-10
Beer, regular (light in color)[‡]	12 oz.	150-190
Beer, light (reduced in calories)	12 oz.	100-145
Wine	5 oz.	120-130
Liquor, 80-proof (gin, rum, whiskey, vodka)	1½ oz.	95-110

*Serving sizes vary. [†]Calories may vary by brand. [‡]Dark beer may have up to 220 calories.
Estimates based on USDA National Nutrient Database for Standard Reference, Release 26, and product labels

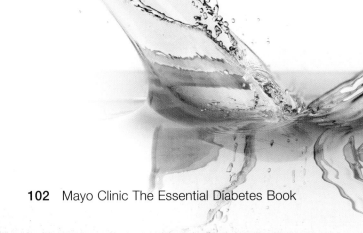

What are your eating triggers?

Does your food record or journal reveal any bad habits? Maybe your problem is your simple love of particular foods, such as ice cream or salty snacks. Or perhaps you have a compulsive need to clean your plate.

To help you be successful in losing weight, you need to identify the factors that lead to your bad habits. Take a few minutes to think about eating triggers and check those that apply to you:

▶ **Time of day.** Are there certain times of the day when you're more inclined to eat?
▶ **Activities.** When you watch TV or read, do you always have food in your hand? Do you eat fast at your desk while you work?
▶ **Foods.** What and how much do you eat? Do you find that the sight or smell of certain foods tempts you to overeat?
▶ **Physical factors.** When you're tired, do you turn to junk food for energy? If you have chronic pain, do you use food to distract you from the pain?
▶ **Emotions.** Do certain feelings, such as stress, cause you to snack endlessly? How do you feel before and after you eat? Do you eat more when you're with certain people? When you're alone?

Addressing your triggers

As you explore solutions, keep these tips in mind:

▶ Avoid keeping unhealthy food in the house or at work. So when you get the urge to eat, you'll grab something healthy.
▶ Limit your time in front of the TV. Keep a glass of water nearby when you're watching TV or reading. If you get hungry, munch on fruits or veggies. Exercise while you're watching TV.
▶ Stay physically active to increase your energy, and get adequate rest.
▶ If coping with pain is an issue, talk with your doctor about pain management strategies.
▶ Do something to distract yourself. Take a walk, listen to music or call a friend. Get support from others.

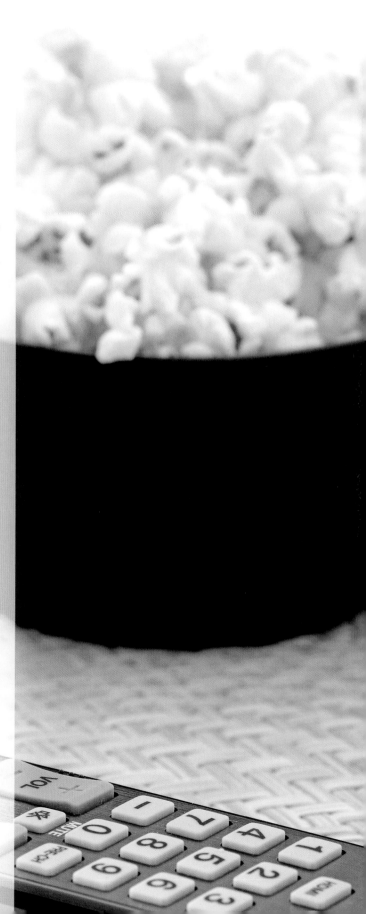

What's your meal routine?

As you examine your eating behaviors and try to identify unhealthy habits, it's important to reflect on your mealtimes. Answer these questions to help assess if your meal routine is helping or hurting your efforts to lose weight. (Snacking isn't considered a meal.)

1. **How many meals do you eat in a day?**

   a. Two or less
   b. Three
   c. Four
   d. Five or more

   Having just one or two meals a day generally isn't the best approach to eating, especially if you're skipping breakfast or snacking throughout the day. When snacking, you probably don't pay attention to how much you eat, and chances are that you'll overeat. Aim for three planned, balanced meals each day.

2. **How many between-meal snacks do you have each day?**

   a. One or none
   b. Two
   c. Three
   d. Four or more

   Snacking between meals to relieve hunger is OK as long as you're nibbling on something healthy. Remember, you can eat unlimited amounts of vegetables and fruits. However, snacks shouldn't take the place of healthy, balanced meals.

3. **Where do you most often eat your meals?**

   a. At the kitchen or dining room table
   b. At the kitchen counter
   c. In another room in the house
   d. On the go, such as in your car or office

   Get into the habit of eating meals at the kitchen or dining room table. Mealtime should be a time to relax and not be rushed or distracted.

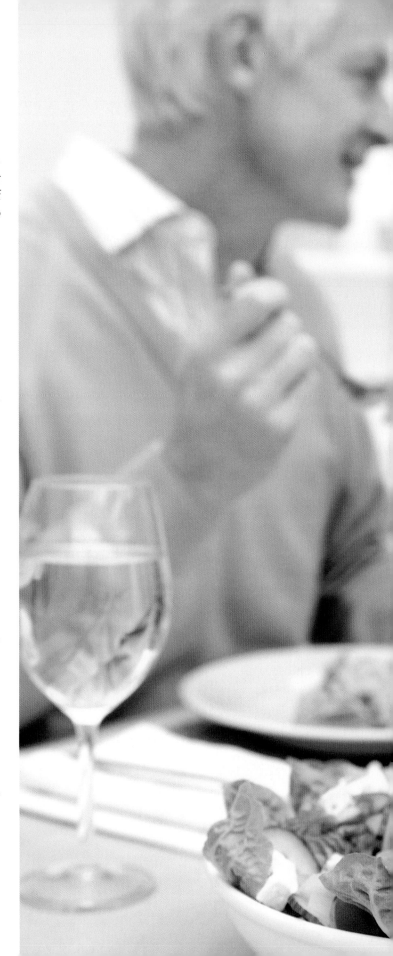

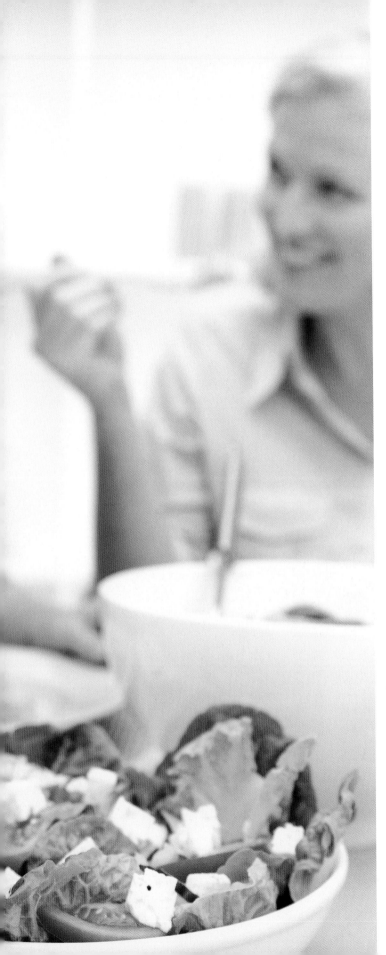

4. **What else are you doing while you're eating?**

   a. Watching a movie or TV
   b. Reading
   c. Preparing food
   d. Sitting at the table and focusing on eating

   Eating while you do other things can be distracting and lead to eating more calories than you intended to. You may even begin to feel the need to eat whenever you do these activities. Break the link — enjoy your food without distraction.

5. **How long does it generally take you to eat a meal?**

   a. Less than five minutes
   b. Five to 10 minutes
   c. 10 to 20 minutes
   d. 20 minutes or more

   The longer it takes you to eat a meal, the more time your brain has to register that you're full. Eating too fast creates a time lag: You overeat before you begin to feel full. Slow down. You'll likely eat less and enjoy the experience more.

Adapting recipes

Many recipes can be modified so that they're healthier. Experiment with some of your favorite recipes using these tips:

- **Reduce the amount of sugar.** You can reduce the amount of sugar in most recipes by one-third to one-half of the original amount without significantly affecting the flavor. Follow the general guideline of a quarter cup of sweetener (sugar, honey or molasses) for every cup of flour.
- **Use less fat.** Fat in many baked products and casseroles can be reduced by one-third to one-half. In baked goods, substitute half the shortening with applesauce or puréed fruit. Look for the words *fat-free* or *low-fat* in products such as milk, yogurt, cheese and spreads.
- **Make substitutions.** In casseroles, cut the amount of meat in half or replace the meat with carrots, onions, lentils or beans. Replace half the flour in baked goods with whole-grain flour.
- **Delete an ingredient.** Eliminate ingredients that are used primarily for appearance or included by habit, such as coconut, frosting and cheese, as well as high-fat or high-sodium condiments such as ketchup, mayonnaise and jam.
- **Reduce your serving size.** Determining a true serving size is half the battle. But sometimes you don't need to eat an entire serving to enjoy a food. By eating half a serving, you consume only half the calories, sugar and fat.
- **Change the method of preparation.** Instead of frying, use low-fat cooking methods, such as baking, broiling, grilling, poaching or steaming.
- **Invest in a good cookbook.** Visit the American Diabetes Association (ADA) website at *www.diabetes.org* to view cookbook titles that are especially helpful for people with diabetes. Also search for "healthy recipes" on *www.MayoClinic.org*.

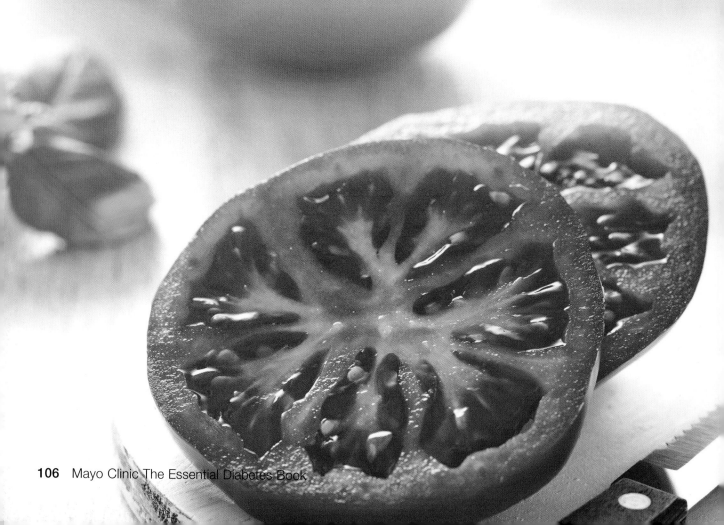

Be a smart shopper

These simple strategies will help ensure that you have the right foods available to follow your healthy-eating plan.

1. Plan ahead

Decide how many major meals you'll be shopping for. Then, consider the number of food items you'll need for breakfasts, lunches and snacks. Take an inventory of your staples, such as low-fat milk, fresh fruits and whole grains.

2. Make a list

A list makes your shopping trip more efficient and helps you avoid impulse purchases, saving both your eating plan and your budget. But don't let your list prevent you from looking for or trying new healthy foods. When making your list, use your weight-loss menus as your guide. Make sure your list includes healthy and convenient snack foods.

3. Shop the perimeter of the store for fresh foods

Chances are that the fresh produce, dairy case, and meat and seafood sections of your grocery store are all located on the perimeter. That's where to focus your shopping when using the Mayo Clinic Healthy Weight Pyramid. Fresh foods are generally better than ready-to-eat foods because they don't contain added sugar, sodium or artificial ingredients, and you can control any ingredients that you add while cooking. Fresh foods also tend to be higher in vitamins, minerals and fiber.

4. Don't shop when hungry

It's harder to resist buying high-fat, high-calorie snack items when you're hungry. So set yourself up for success and shop after you've eaten a good meal. If you do find yourself shopping on an empty stomach, drink some water or buy a piece of fruit to munch on to avoid unhealthy impulse buys.

5. Read nutrition labels

Check nutrition labels for serving size, fat, cholesterol and sodium, in particular. Remember, even low-fat and fat-free foods can pack a lot of calories. Don't be fooled. The label will list the calories, fat, cholesterol and sodium for one serving — but keep in mind that you might eat more than one serving at a time. Compare similar products so that you can choose the healthiest.

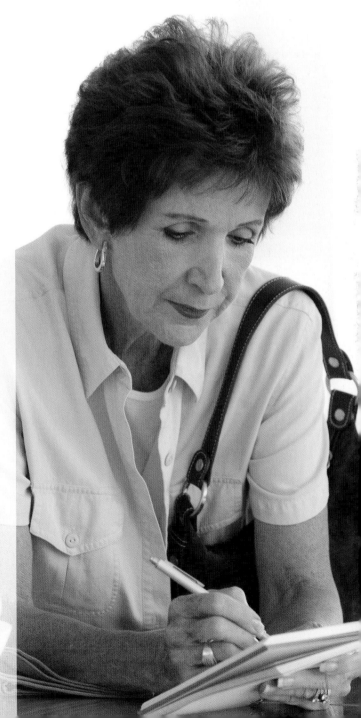

Willpower vs. self-control

You may think that you can reach a healthy weight if you exert enough willpower. You just won't eat those foods that cause you to gain weight. Unfortunately, this can set you up to fail as your willpower inevitably cracks. This is when many people give up. "I already broke the rules, so I might as well keep eating." Don't be so hard on yourself. Be realistic — make healthy behavior choices easier through planning, so you can rely on self-control instead of willpower. These examples show the difference:

Willpower	Self-control
I'll make a cheesecake for the family, but I won't eat any of it.	I won't make a cheesecake, but I can have an occasional slice when I dine out.
We'll go to the buffet, but I'll just have salad.	We'll go to a restaurant that offers small portions and low-fat or vegetarian items.
I'll bring my favorite chocolate dessert for my co-workers, but I won't have any of it.	I'll bring a tasty healthy dessert for my co-workers so that I can have some, too.

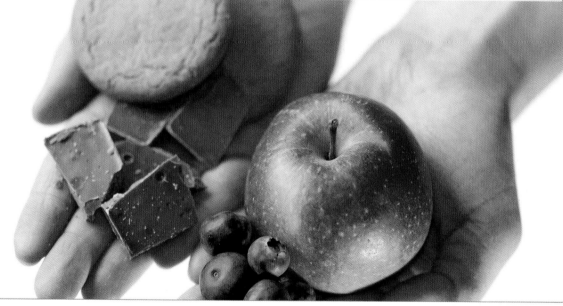

Is it OK to drink liquid meal replacement products in place of meals if I don't have time to eat?

While a healthy diet that includes whole grains, fruits and vegetables is best, a meal replacement product is a convenient alternative when eating a healthy meal isn't possible. Most meal replacement products, such as a shake or meal bar, provide fewer than 400 calories a meal and are fortified with vitamins and minerals. Ask your doctor or dietitian if meal replacement products fit into your specific meal planning.

Bumps in the road: Overcoming setbacks

It's inevitable that you'll have setbacks, and that's OK. But don't use your setbacks as an excuse to dump your eating goals. Instead, renew your determination and simply continue on with your plan. For example, if you ate a rich dessert that you hadn't planned on, think about what triggered you to do so and try to learn from it.

Getting back on track

Use the following tips to help you get back on track after a setback.

Take charge

Accept responsibility for your own behavior. Remember that ultimately only you can help yourself lose weight.

Avoid risky situations

If all-you-can-eat buffets are just too tempting, avoid them — at least until you feel more in control of your new eating behavior.

Think it through

If you're tempted to indulge in an old favorite food, first ask yourself if you're really hungry. Chances are, it's a craving and you may be able to talk yourself out of it. If not, wait a few minutes and see if the desire passes. Or try distracting yourself from your urge to eat — call a friend or take the dog for a walk. If the craving still doesn't pass, have a glass of water and a piece of fruit instead.

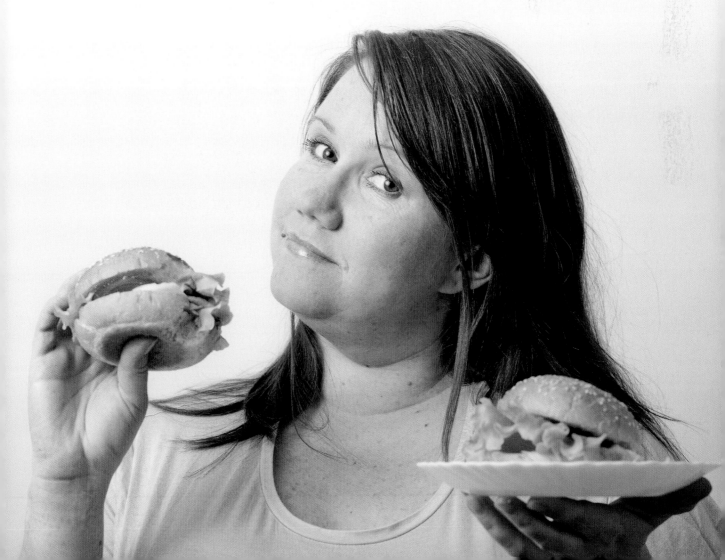

Be gentle with yourself

Practice self-forgiveness. Don't let negative self-talk ("I've blown it now!") get in your way of getting back on track with your eating goals. Try not to think of your slip-up as a catastrophe. Remember that mistakes happen and that each day is a chance to start anew.

Ask for and accept support

Accepting support from others isn't a sign of weakness, nor does it mean that you're failing. Asking for support is a sign of good judgment. You need support from others to help keep you on track.

Find healthy ways to deal with stress

There are many self-help strategies to deal with stress. Perhaps you need to manage your time better or learn to say no if your schedule is overloaded. You might want to learn relaxation techniques, such as deep breathing or meditation. Make sure you get enough sleep and set aside at least one night each week for recreation. Go for a swim or play golf with friends. You also might consider taking a stress management class. Don't be afraid to seek professional help if needed.

Plan your strategy

Clearly identify the problem, and then create a list of possible solutions. Try a solution. If it works, you've got a strategy for preventing another lapse. If it doesn't, try the next solution and keep trying until you find one that works.

Re-evaluate your goals

Your weight-loss goals may change over time. Review them periodically and make certain they're still realistic. Change them as needed. Remember, healthy weight loss comes gradually — 1 or 2 pounds a week.

Although setbacks are disappointing, they can help you learn to keep your goals realistic, what high-risk situations to avoid, or what certain strategies don't work for you.

Above all, realize that you're not a failure. Reverting to old behaviors doesn't mean that all hope is lost. It just means that you need to recharge your motivation, recommit to your program and return to healthy behaviors.

Habits for a lifetime

It takes time and regular reinforcement for your new healthy behaviors to become habits. Eventually you'll know how to identify healthy foods, determine a serving and calculate how many servings you need. Also strive to make physical activity and exercise a daily routine. Once these become habits, you're on your way to maintaining a healthy weight for life.

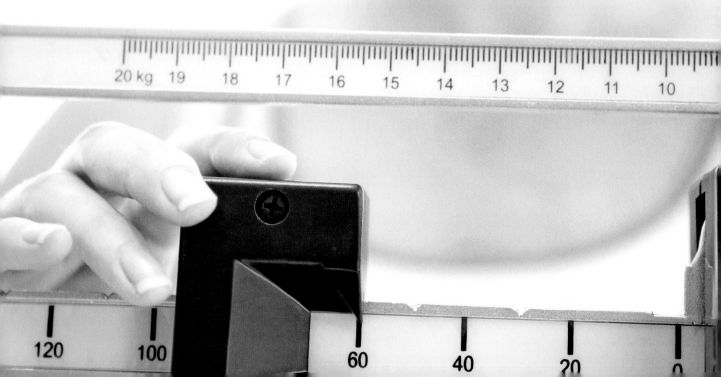

Use whatever works

If you favor computers, tablet or mobile apps, or other technical tools, use them to your advantage. Use whatever devices or functions — trackers, reminders or alarms — that can help you meet your goals.

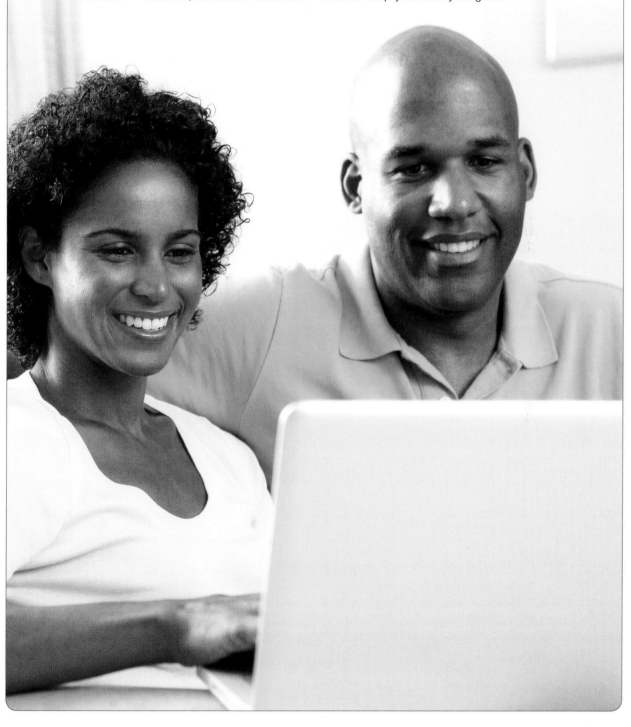

Chapter 5
Getting More Active

Physical activity vs. exercise 114

Fitness is essential to your health 115

Create a personal fitness plan 117

Tackle your exercise barriers 120

Aerobic exercise 122

Walking to better health 124

Staying hydrated 128

How much exercise? 129

Stretching exercises 130

Strengthening exercises 132

Avoiding injury 135

Exercise and regular monitoring 136

Getting and staying motivated 137

Fitness for kids 140

A visit with Paula Ricke

"Research shows that physical activity is important when it comes to management of diabetes. Physical activity can help lower your blood sugar (glucose) as well as improve your body's ability to use insulin."

You may have heard it before, and it's true. Research shows that physical activity is important when it comes to management of diabetes. Physical activity can help lower your blood sugar (glucose) as well as improve your body's ability to use insulin. There are numerous other benefits, such as help with weight loss, reduction in stress levels, a lower risk of heart disease or stroke, and much more.

If you're thinking, "That sounds great, but I don't have time to be active," you're not alone. Time is the No. 1 barrier to being physically active. Being healthy and fit doesn't mean hours of activity each day; it simply means moving more. Find simple ways to build activity into your day. Try walking as you talk on the phone, playing with your children, carrying your own groceries or moving during commercial breaks. Be creative and do what works for you.

In combination with daily physical activity, work toward engaging in aerobic activity. Aerobic activity is a planned session of activity in which the heart rate is elevated. Examples include walking at a moderate pace or swimming laps. Your goal is to work up to 30 minutes of physical activity at least five days a week. The activity doesn't have to be a consecutive 30 minutes to be beneficial. Three 10-minute bouts of activity spaced throughout your day will give you the same benefit.

The first step is the hardest, and if you're reading this, you've already started to take that first step. Good for you. Next, ask yourself these two questions: What can I do to be physically active today? What am I ready for? Answer these questions and then fill in the blank: Today I will _____ to be active. No one can tell you what's best for you; only you can determine that. Start slow and go one day at a time.

One way to help ensure your success is to write SMART goals. SMART goals are specific, measurable, attainable, relevant and time-limited. If your goal is to

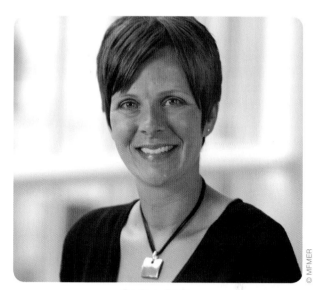

Paula L. Ricke
Exercise Specialist
Dan Abraham Healthy Living Center

take a walk three times a week, that's great, but how are you going to achieve this goal? By adjusting your goal to say, "I am going to walk the trail outside my office for 30 minutes over my lunch hour on Tuesday, Thursday and Friday," you've created a SMART goal. The key is to make your goals an obtainable challenge and to avoid the all-or-nothing thinking.

Talk with your doctor before starting a physical activity program. Ask if there's a need to change any medicines, how often you should check your blood glucose and if there are exercises you should avoid based on your past health history. Once you have met with your health care team, you are ready to move forward.

In this chapter you will learn more about the benefits of being physically active in managing diabetes, how to get started with an activity program as well as other tips to help you increase your personal success. Remember, being physically active and taking care of yourself are for you. Taking time to be healthy is not selfish; it's simply a must. Take time to write down your goals and develop your physical activity plan today. Your body will thank you for it.

Our bodies are designed to move, even if modern society makes it easy to do anything but that. You may sit at a desk all day and then come home and watch TV or put your feet up and read.

It takes a special effort to incorporate exercise and other physical activity into your day. But that effort brings a bounty of health benefits — especially if you have diabetes.

The information in this chapter can help you get started on the road to a more active life. You don't have to knock yourself out to reap the benefits. Increased physical activity and a moderate amount of exercise can improve your fitness and help control your diabetes.

Physical activity vs. exercise

Physical activity refers to any body movement that burns calories, such as mowing the lawn, doing housework or climbing stairs.

Exercise is a more structured form of physical activity. It involves a series of repetitive movements designed to strengthen or develop some part of your body or improve your cardiovascular fitness. Exercise includes walking, swimming, bicycling and many other activities.

Whether you're exercising or doing other types of physical activity, monitor your blood sugar (glucose) level and adjust your medications so that your glucose doesn't drop too low.

Every move counts

Regular exercise provides the greatest reward for your efforts, but you also can enjoy health benefits simply by moving around more during the day.

Regular physical activity also helps lower your blood glucose, as well as your blood cholesterol and blood pressure.

Look for ways to build more physical activity into your day Here are a few easy suggestions at home, the office, and out and about:

- ▌ Take the stairs instead of the elevator.
- ▌ Park farther from work and walk.
- ▌ Wash your car instead of taking it to the carwash.
- ▌ Walk or bike short distances instead of driving.
- ▌ Take walks with your family to explore your neighborhood.
- ▌ Walk your dog more often.
- ▌ Sweep the floors, patio and front sidewalk every day.
- ▌ Work in your garden.
- ▌ Get up to change channels on your TV instead of using the remote control.

Pedometers: Step up your health

If you need motivation to get moving, consider buying a pedometer. This small, inexpensive device detects body motion, counts steps and displays the number on a small screen. Many pedometers have additional features.

Set your pedometer goals based on your fitness level and track your progress. Gradually work your way up to at least 10,000 steps a day.

Choose a pedometer that:
- ▌ Is simple to use and easy to read
- ▌ Can be read in indoor and outdoor lighting
- ▌ Is lightweight and fits snugly on your clothes
- ▌ Has a sturdy clip and a security strap so that you won't lose it

Keep in mind that a pedometer may record other movements you make (not just walking) as steps taken, making the total count at the end of the day a bit high.

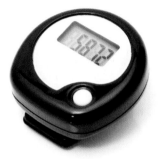

Fitness is essential to your health

By increasing your daily physical activity and getting a moderate amount of exercise, you can significantly improve your health and well-being.

Among other benefits, regular physical activity can help prevent or manage:

▶ Diabetes
▶ Coronary artery disease
▶ High blood pressure
▶ Stroke
▶ Osteoporosis
▶ Colon cancer
▶ Depression

It may sound simplistic, but 30 minutes of physical activity a day can do you a world of good. Even if you do 10 minutes of physical activity three times a day, you'll still get health benefits.

You can do it!

If you think physical activity and exercise are difficult because you don't have time, start gradually. Get more physically active with common activities, such as household chores, walking the dog, washing your car or raking your yard.

If you have health problems, get creative. Medical research shows that physical activity is both safe and beneficial for people with arthritis, osteoporosis and other chronic conditions. In fact, lack of physical activity and exercise can make your condition worse — or at least more difficult to live with.

If you have arthritis, for instance, consider water exercise. Ask your doctor or physical therapist what might work best for you. Starting a fitness program is an important decision, but it doesn't have to be overwhelming. By planning carefully and pacing yourself, you can establish a healthy habit that lasts a lifetime.

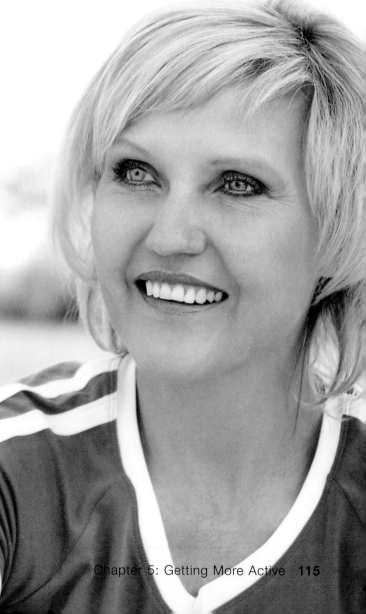

How fit are you?

To assess how fit you are, circle the point value (1, 2 or 3) for each question. Add up the points.

Do you have enough energy to do the things you like to do?
1. Rarely or never
2. Sometimes
3. Always or most of the time

Do you have enough stamina and strength to carry out the daily tasks of your life?
1. Rarely or never
2. Sometimes
3. Always or most of the time

Can you walk a mile without feeling winded or fatigued?
1. No
2. Sometimes
3. Yes

Can you climb two flights of stairs without feeling winded or fatigued?
1. No
2. Sometimes
3. Yes

Can you do at least five pushups before you need to stop for a rest?
1. No
2. Sometimes
3. Yes

Can you touch your toes while standing?
1. No
2. Sometimes
3. Yes

Can you carry on a conversation while doing light to moderate activities, such as brisk walking?
1. No
2. Sometimes
3. Yes

About how many days a week do you get at least 30 minutes of moderately vigorous activity, such as hiking or biking?
1. Two days or fewer
2. Three or four days
3. Five to seven days

About how many days a week do you get at least 20 minutes of vigorous activity, such as jogging, participating in a cardio class or playing singles tennis?
1. None
2. One to three days
3. Four or more days

About how many minutes do you walk during the day, including doing chores around the house, walking from your car to the office or store, or doing errands at work?
1. Less than 30 minutes
2. 30 to 60 minutes
3. More than 60 minutes

How did you score?

Total score:

▶ **10 to 19 points.** For fitness and health benefits, look for ways to get in 30 minutes or more of physical activity most days, even if it's just 10 minutes at a time.
▶ **20 to 25 points.** You're on the right track, but your activity level could use a boost. Look for ways to add more activity to your day or increase the intensity.
▶ **26 to 30 points.** Way to go! You're well on your way to maintaining overall fitness. Keep up the good work!

Create a personal fitness plan

The challenge of any fitness plan is to create a plan that's varied and lively — one that will become a healthy and fun habit for a lifetime. That means creating your own personal plan and getting a host of health benefits.

The sooner you start, the less you'll need to worry about later. For a fitness program to work, it's important to:

▶ Assess your fitness
▶ Get motivated
▶ Keep physically active
▶ Choose activities that you enjoy
▶ Plan your exercise routine
▶ Include variety

Make fitness activities a priority in your schedule. And remember any movement counts. Do things that you enjoy. Dance, ride a bike or take a brisk walk on a nature trail. Do a home workout using a fitness DVD.

Getting motivated

For most people, getting started on a fitness program is the hardest step. Start by creating an action plan.

Recognize what does or doesn't motivate you. What can you do differently to help you succeed this time? What past successes have you had?

Ask for support. Who can you exercise with or who can support you in other ways?

Focus on the process and take small steps. Set realistic, attainable goals. Assess them and change them if needed.

Monitor your progress. Keep track of your progress as you go along.

Staying motivated

To stay committed to your plan:

▶ **Expand your definition of fitness activity.** It's not just working out in the gym — it's any physical activity.

▶ **Experiment and find fitness activities that you enjoy.** You're more likely to stick with your fitness plan if you have fun doing it.
▶ **Make a commitment and don't look too far ahead.** What can you do today to make this fitness plan work for you?
▶ **Practice positive self-talk.** Positive self-talk can increase your energy, motivation and positive attitude, while negative self-talk is critical and anxiety producing. Become aware of what you're saying to yourself and make it more positive. For example, instead of telling yourself "I'm too tired to exercise," say "I'm going to feel more energized after exercising."

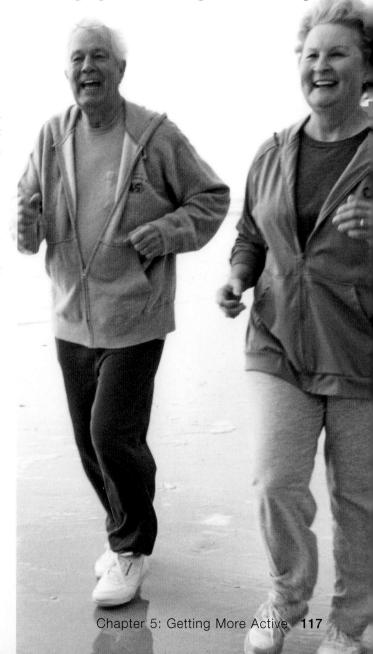

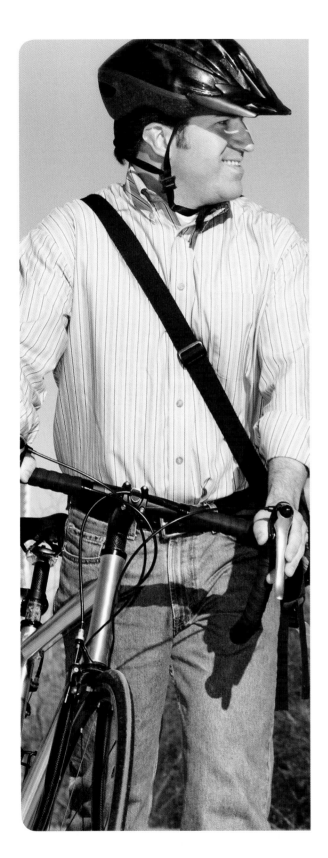

Keeping physically active

The key to staying physically active is making it convenient. There are tips that can help at home and at work.

Make the most of your time at home

To fit physical activity into your home life:

- **Wake up early.** Get up 30 minutes earlier than you normally do and use the additional time to walk on your treadmill or take a brisk walk around the neighborhood.
- **Make household chores count.** Mop the floor, scrub the tub, mow the lawn with a push mower or do other chores at a pace fast enough to get your heart pumping.
- **Be active while watching TV.** Use hand weights, ride a stationary bike or do a stretching routine during your favorite shows.
- **Involve the whole family.** Take group walks before or after dinner. Play catch. Ride your bikes.
- **Get your dog into the act.** Take daily walks with Fido. If you don't have a dog, offer to walk your neighbor's dog.

Work out at work

To fit in more physical activity while you're on the job:

- **Schedule physical activity as an appointment.** Don't change your plans for physical activity unless you absolutely have to — this is important to your health.
- **Make the most of your commute.** Walk or bike to work. If you ride the bus, get off a few blocks early and walk the rest of the way.
- **Take the stairs.** If you have a meeting on another floor, get off the elevator a few floors early and use the stairs. Better yet, skip the elevator entirely.
- **Take fitness breaks.** Rather than hanging out in the lounge and having coffee or a snack, take a short walk.
- **Start a lunchtime walking group with your co-workers.** The regular routine and support of your co-workers may help you stick with the program.
- **If you travel for work, keep physically active.** Choose a hotel with a fitness facility or just get out and walk when you have time.

Choose activities that you enjoy

Exercise is more fun when you enjoy what you're doing. Look at all of the options available to you. What would you like to do or like to learn?

Going solo
You might enjoy these activities if you're looking to be active on your own:
- Aerobics
- Bicycling — stationary or outdoors
- Canoeing, kayaking or rowing
- Hiking or walking
- Jogging or running
- Jumping rope
- Pilates
- Skating: ice or in-line
- Skiing — cross-country, downhill or ski machine
- Snowshoeing
- Swimming
- Weightlifting
- Yoga

With a friend
Try any of the activities with a friend or you might consider:
- Badminton
- Dancing
- Frisbee golf
- Golfing
- Playing catch
- Playing frisbee
- Racquetball
- Squash
- Table tennis
- Tandem bicycling
- Tennis
- Video games that require physical activity

A class
For a more structured approach, try a class:
- Aerobics
- Dancing
- Jazzercise
- Kickboxing
- Martial arts
- Pilates
- Rock climbing
- Spinning (indoor cycling)
- Tai chi
- Water aerobics
- Yoga

A team
The camaraderie of team sports may help keep you motivated:
- Baseball
- Basketball
- Bowling
- Football
- Hockey — field or ice
- Lacrosse
- Rugby
- Soccer
- Softball
- Tennis
- Ultimate frisbee
- Volleyball

Tackle your exercise barriers

Getting started with an exercise routine can be difficult. But if you want to stay healthy, you need to get past those barriers that are preventing you from making exercise a daily habit.

Barriers	Possible solutions
❏ Lack of time	› Break the activity into shorter periods, such as 10-minute walks. › Identify time wasters, such as watching TV. › Schedule exercise into your daily routine. › Reframe your concept of exercise to include everyday activities.
❏ Boredom	› Change your routine periodically. › Do a variety of activities rather than one or two. › Exercise with a friend or in a group. › Join a health club or take a fitness class. › Listen to music or watch TV while you work out. › Challenge yourself with new goals. › Get a new gadget or piece of equipment.
❏ Inconvenience	› Work out at home rather than at a club. › Choose activities that require minimal equipment and facilities. › Incorporate physical activity into your daily routine. › Choose activities that don't depend on good weather or daylight.
❏ Age	› You're never too old to exercise. Exercise provides benefits to all ages, and it may prevent, delay or improve diseases as you get older.
❏ Obesity	› Athletes may appear slim, trim and toned. But if you look around, you'll see that few people who exercise have a perfect body. Walkers, bicyclers and golfers come in all shapes and sizes.
❏ Injury	› Warm up and cool down when you exercise. › Talk to your doctor about appropriate exercise for your age, fitness level, skill level and health status. › Choose low-risk activities. › Use the proper equipment and dress for the weather conditions.

Barriers	Possible solutions
❑ Travel	› Find out what fitness facilities, parks or waking paths are available where you're going. › Walk around the airport terminal. › Stretch and walk during your flight, or take short walking breaks during a road trip. › Choose a hotel with fitness equipment or a pool, or walk the halls and climb the stairs in your hotel.
❑ Lack of facilities or resources	› Select activities you can do on your own, such as walking, jogging or jumping rope. › Identify inexpensive, convenient community resources, such as park and recreation centers or community education programs.
❑ Illness	› You don't want to exercise if your blood glucose is out of control. But simply having diabetes isn't a reason to avoid exercise. Just the opposite — it's a reason to exercise. › Avoid strenuous exercise when you're sick. But you may be able to work out at a reduced intensity.
❑ Weather	› Choose activities that you can do regardless of the weather, such as indoor cycling, aerobics, indoor swimming, dancing or mall walking.
❑ Lifestyle changes	› During stressful times, consider a moderate program of physical activity.
❑ Overtraining	› Learn the signs of overtraining. › Vary your activities, as well as their order and intensity. › Increase the length and intensity of your workouts gradually. › Build light workouts and rest days into your schedule. › Be sure to get adequate nutrition and sleep.

Aerobic exercise

Aerobic exercise improves the health of your heart, lungs and circulatory system. Aerobic means "with oxygen." Aerobic activities increase your breathing and heart rate.

Keep in mind that aerobic activities are endurance activities that don't require excessive speed. For an activity to be aerobic, it should be performed at a low to moderate intensity level. Aerobic activities should make up the core of your exercise program. Examples of aerobic activities include:

▶ Walking
▶ Cross-country skiing
▶ Jogging
▶ Skating
▶ Bicycling
▶ Dancing
▶ Tennis
▶ Cardio classes
▶ Swimming

A higher aerobic capacity improves your endurance, making it easier for you to do household chores and climb stairs without shortness of breath.

Getting started

These tips can help you incorporate aerobic activity into your daily schedule:

▶ A beginning goal is to exercise at least three days a week and work up to five days a week.
▶ Before doing any aerobic activity, warm up for at least five minutes.
▶ Work toward a goal of exercising for 30 to 60 minutes daily. This can be done continuously or divided into shorter sessions throughout the day.
▶ Spend at least five minutes cooling down at the end of your workout.
▶ Try to increase your level of physical activity every day, even if it's not a scheduled exercise day. Jog in place while waiting for the bus or park a few blocks away from your meeting place and walk.

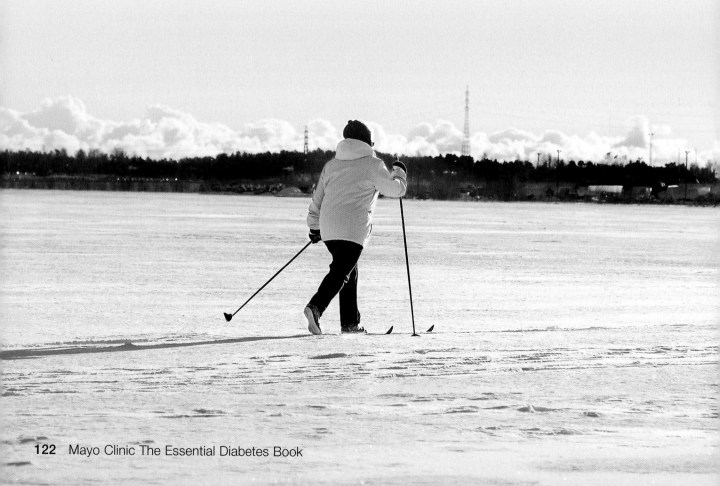

Gauging exercise intensity

When you're doing physical activity, exercise intensity correlates with how hard the activity feels to you. Exercise intensity is also reflected in how hard your heart is working. Here are some clues to help you judge your exercise intensity:

Light exercise intensity
▶ You have no noticeable changes in your breathing pattern
▶ You don't break a sweat (unless it's very hot or humid)
▶ You can easily carry on a full conversation or even sing

Moderate exercise intensity
▶ Your breathing quickens, but you're not out of breath
▶ You develop a light sweat after about 10 minutes of activity
▶ You can carry on a conversation, but you can't sing

Vigorous exercise intensity
▶ Your breathing is deep and rapid
▶ You develop a sweat after a few minutes of activity
▶ You can't say more than a few words without pausing for breath

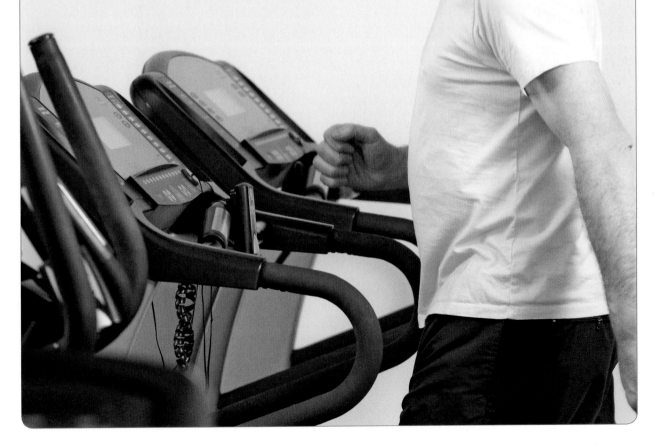

Walking shoes: Features and fit

Wearing walking shoes that are comfortable and fit properly can help prevent blisters, calluses and other injuries. Use this checklist to help make your decision:

▶ Consider buying shoes at an athletic store with professional shoe fitters.

▶ Wear the same socks you'll wear when walking.

▶ Ask the salesperson to measure both feet and help determine your foot type (normal, flat or high arches).

▶ If one foot is larger than the other is, buy shoes to fit your larger foot.

▶ Wiggle your toes to be sure you have at least a quarter-inch space after your longest toe.

▶ Be sure the shoe is wide enough. The width and heel should be snug, but not tight.

▶ If you can detect the outline of your toes in the top or on the side of the shoe, try a larger size or wider shoe.

▶ Walk in the shoes before buying them. They should feel comfortable right away.

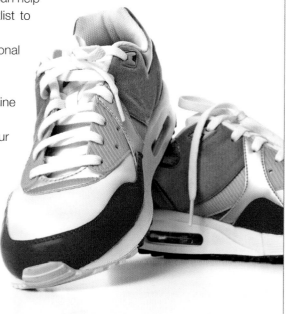

Walking to better health

Walking is a low-impact activity that can deliver many of the benefits of aerobic exercise. It's safe, simple and has many health benefits.

Benefits of walking

Walking on a regular basis is beneficial to many aspects of your health. It can help:

▶ Reduce your risk of type 2 diabetes
▶ Manage your diabetes
▶ Reduce your risk of a heart attack
▶ Prevent or reduce high blood pressure
▶ Manage your weight
▶ Manage stress and boost your spirits
▶ Maintain bone density
▶ Stay strong and active

Prepare yourself
To prevent pain and injury, prepare yourself for walking.

Wear walking shoes and appropriate clothing
Select comfortable footwear that fits properly. Your walking shoes should be of good quality and fit you well. Wear loose-fitting, comfortable clothing and dress in layers if you need to adjust to changing temperatures. Avoid rubberized materials, as they don't allow perspiration to evaporate. Wear bright colors or reflective tape after dark so motorists can see you.

Warm up
Spend about five minutes walking slowly to warm up your muscles. You can walk in place if you want. Increase your pace until you feel warm. Warming up your muscles reduces your risk of injury.

Stretch
After warming up, stretch your muscles for about five minutes.

Getting started

There are steps you can take to help ensure your walking success.

Start slow and easy

Unless you're a seasoned walker, it's best to start slow and easy. At first, walk only as far or fast as you find comfortable. For example, if you can walk for only a few minutes, try short daily sessions of three to five minutes and slowly build up to 15 minutes twice a week. Then, over several weeks' time, you can gradually work your way up to 30 minutes of walking five days a week.

Use proper technique to avoid injury and setbacks

If your posture is poor or your movements are exaggerated, you increase your risk of injury.

Measure the intensity of your workout

If you're so out of breath that you can't carry on a conversation, you're probably walking too fast and should slow down.

Track your progress

Keep a record of how many steps you take or miles you walk and how long it takes so that you can track your progress. Record these numbers in a walking journal or on a computer spreadsheet.

You can also keep track of your steps or miles by wearing a pedometer (see page 114) or a device that uses satellite technology and allows you to download data to a computer, or by using a pedometer app with your cellphone.

Stay motivated

To stay motivated, be patient and flexible with yourself. If you don't meet your daily goal one day, do the best you can, then get back to your regular walking routine the next day. Remember how good it feels after you've had a refreshing walk.

Plan several different routes for variety, and make walking fun — a great way is to invite friends, family or co-workers to join you. Once you take that first step, you're on your way to an important destination — better health.

Try this 10-week walking schedule

Are you looking to ease into getting in shape? This 10-week walking schedule can start you on the path to better fitness and health.

Week	Walking schedule*	Weekly total (time x days a week)†
1	15 minutes, 2 days	30 minutes
2	15 minutes, 3 days	45 minutes
3	20 minutes, 3 days	60 minutes
4	25 minutes, 3 days	75 minutes
5 & 6	30 minutes, 3 days	90 minutes
7 & 8	30 minutes, 4 days	120 minutes
9 & 10	30 minutes, 5 days	150 minutes

*Before starting this walking schedule, you may need to talk with your doctor.   †Doesn't include warm-up and cool-down time.

What the research shows

Guidelines published by the American Association of Clinical Endocrinologists note that walking just 40 minutes four times a week is enough to lower insulin resistance, improving blood glucose control. In addition, an eight-year study of more than 70,000 women suggests that one hour a day of brisk walking may cut a woman's risk of developing type 2 diabetes almost in half.

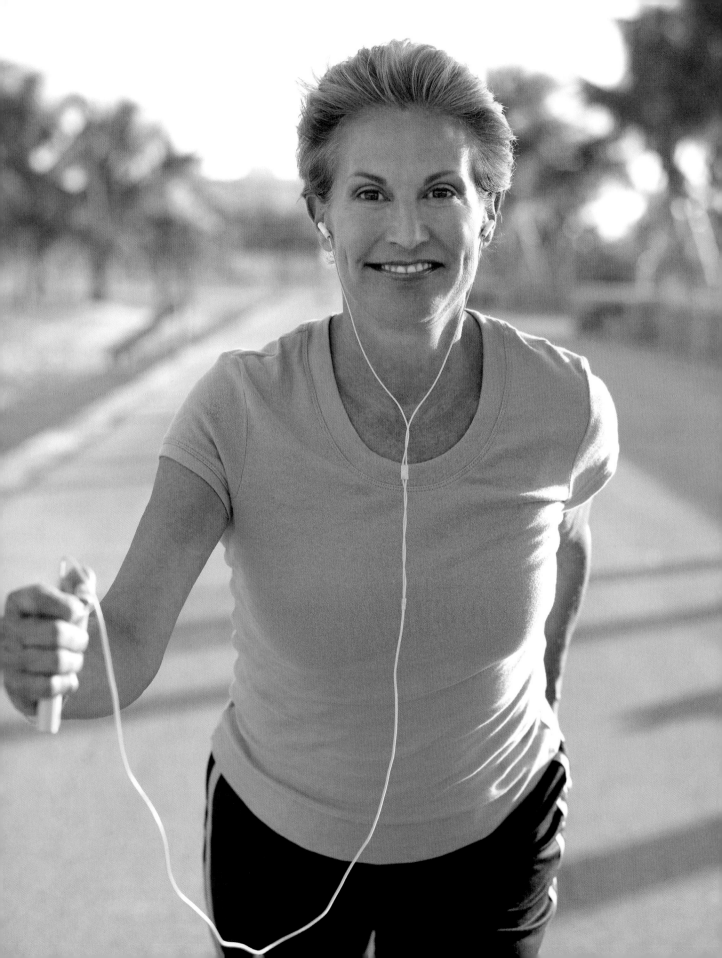

Calories burned in 1 hour

This chart shows the estimated number of calories burned while performing a number of activities for one hour at a moderately intense level.

If your weight range isn't shown, you can use this formula:
1. Find an activity in the chart.
2. Take the maximum number of calories burned from the column for a 170- to 180-pound person.
3. Multiply this by your weight.
4. Divide by 175.

For example, if you weigh 220 pounds and jog 5 mph, here's the calculation:

$$\frac{656 \times 220}{175} = 825 \text{ calories in 1 hour}$$

Moderately intense activity (1 hour)	Calories burned		Moderately intense activity (1 hour)	Calories burned	
	140 to 150 Lb. person	170 to 180 Lb. person		140 to 150 Lb. person	170 to 180 Lb. person
Aerobic dancing	416–442	501–533	Jumping rope	640–680	770–820
Backpacking	448–476	539–574	Racquetball	448–476	539–574
Badminton	288–306	347–369	Running, 8 mph	864–918	1,040–1,107
Bicycling (outdoor)	512–544	616–656	Skating (ice or in-line)	448–476	539–574
Bicycling (stationary)	448–476	539–574	Skiing (cross-country)	512–544	616–656
Bowling	192–204	231–246	Skiing (downhill)	384–408	462–492
Canoeing	224–238	270–287	Stair climbing	576–612	693–738
Dancing	288–306	347–369	Swimming	384–408	462–492
Gardening	256–272	308–328	Tennis	448–476	539–574
Golfing (carrying bag)	288–306	347–369	Volleyball	192–204	231–246
Hiking	384–408	462–492	Walking, 2 mph	160–170	193–2050
Jogging, 5 mph	512–544	616–656	Walking, 3.5 mph	243–258	293–312

Staying hydrated

When you exercise, you need extra water to maintain your normal body temperature and cool working muscles. To help replace fluid lost through perspiration, drink water before and after physical activity.

If you take a brisk walk for more than 45 minutes, drink water every 15 to 20 minutes, especially in hot weather. To avoid dehydration, water is best. You don't need sports drinks except for long or intense exercise.

You're likely well-hydrated if the color of your urine is clear or light. But if your urine is a dark yellow or amber color, you may not be getting enough water. Drinking plenty of water is essential to good health.

Here's why you need lots of water every day:

▶ Regulates body temperature
▶ Moistens tissues such as those in the mouth, eyes and nose
▶ Lubricates joints
▶ Protects body organs and tissues
▶ Helps prevent constipation
▶ Carries nutrients and oxygen to the cells of your body
▶ Lessens the burden on the kidneys and liver by flushing out waste products
▶ Helps dissolve minerals and other nutrients to make them accessible to the body

Energy & sports drinks

Some energy and sports drinks may be useful in certain circumstances — but others may actually be harmful. Here's a brief summary:

▶ **Energy drinks.** These drinks typically contain a lot of carbohydrates, caffeine and other stimulants. Carbohydrates can boost energy, but too much caffeine or other stimulants can make your heart beat faster, raise your blood pressure, and cause nervousness, irritability and insomnia.

▶ **Sports drinks.** These products, such as All Sport, Gatorade and Powerade, typically contain carbohydrates and electrolytes, which can increase energy and replace minerals lost during sweat. Sports drinks may help if you've exercised for 90 minutes, or for 60 minutes if your activity is particularly intense or it's very hot. Beware of products that offer extra ingredients to improve performance — they can be risky.

▶ **Fitness water.** This water has some vitamins, minerals, carbohydrates, flavoring and sometimes caffeine. There's little, if any, added value of nutrients in the amounts supplied. But if you like them, just avoid the products with caffeine.

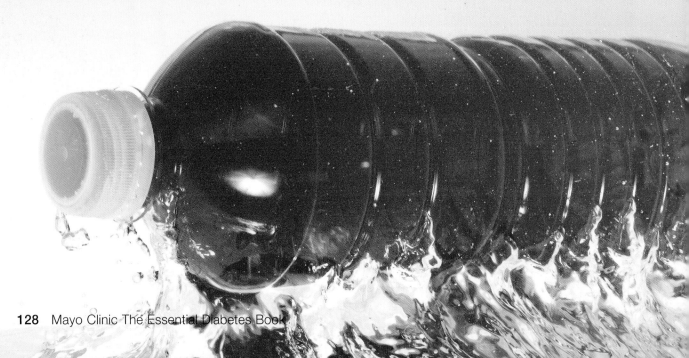

How much exercise?

The answer to this question varies — and will change over the course of your lifetime.

Essentially, the amount of exercise you need is based on some widely accepted guidelines and your specific goals.

Many health agencies and organizations recommend that for general health and well-being, adults should get 30 minutes of moderate activity at least five days a week. Children and teens should get 60 minutes of physical activity a day.

A bit of a controversy occurred in 2002 when the Institute of Medicine (IOM) issued a report recommending that adults spend at least 60 minutes in moderately intense physical activity every day.

Why is the IOM's recommendation higher? The unfortunate trend is that Americans are getting heavier. And evidence shows that 30 minutes of activity most days of the week may not be enough for some people to maintain a healthy weight. The IOM factored this trend into its recommendation.

The bottom line is this: It's apparent that 30 minutes of physical activity most days of the week will deliver health benefits. Getting 60 minutes of activity, on the other hand, will deliver greater benefits — and may be necessary to avoid weight gain.

Build up gradually

If you haven't been active for a long time, start slowly and gradually build up your endurance. Begin by exercising 10 minutes a day. Each week, increase the length of time you exercise by five minutes, and keep adding increments.

To improve your total fitness, stretch for a few minutes after aerobic exercise to increase the flexibility in your muscles and the range of motion of your joints. Also, combine aerobic activity with strengthening exercises about two days a week.

If you don't have 30 minutes or more to exercise, it's OK to break your routine into shorter intervals. For example. you might ride a stationary bicycle for

Warning signs: When to stop

Moderate physical activity should cause you to breathe faster and feel like you're working. But if you experience any of these signs or symptoms during exercise, stop immediately and seek medical attention:

▶ Chest pain or tightness
▶ Dizziness or faintness
▶ Pain in an arm or your jaw
▶ Severe shortness of breath
▶ Excessive fatigue
▶ Bursts of very rapid or slow heart rate
▶ An irregular heartbeat
▶ Severe joint or muscle pain
▶ Joint swelling

10 to 15 minutes in the morning before going to work, walk for 10 to 15 minutes during your lunch hour and do strengthening exercises for 10 to 15 minutes in the evening.

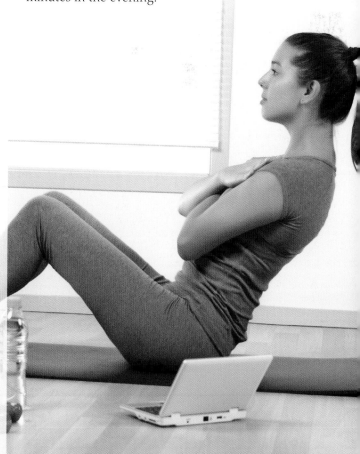

Stretching exercises

Stretching before and after aerobic activity helps increase the range of motion around your joints and helps prevent joint pain and injury.

But don't stretch a "cold" muscle: If you stretch before you exercise, do a short three- to five-minute warm-up first, such as low-intensity walking. If you only have time to stretch once, stretch after you exercise, when your muscles are warmed up. Stretch slowly and gently, only until you feel slight tension in your muscles.

Here are four stretches. Stretch each muscle group once. Try to do them three to five days a week and after physical activity.

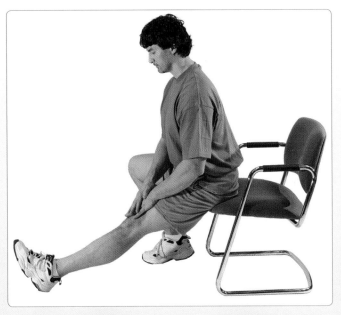

Seated hamstring stretch
Sit on a sturdy chair as shown. Maintain your normal back arch. Slowly straighten your left knee until you feel a stretch in the back of your thigh (hamstring). You may apply gentle downward pressure with your hands. Hold for 30 seconds. Relax. Repeat with the other leg.

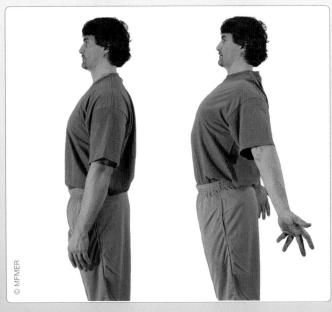

Chest stretch
Stand with arms at your sides. Then move your arms backward while rotating your palms forward as shown at right. Squeeze your shoulder blades together, breathe deeply and lift your chest upward. Hold for 30 seconds while breathing freely, then relax. Return to starting position. Repeat.

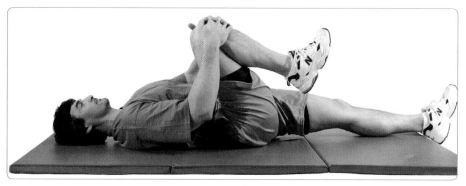

Knee-to-chest stretch*

Lie on a firm surface with your right knee bent (heel flat on the surface) and your left leg straight — or keep both knees bent if that's more comfortable. Gently pull the right knee toward your right shoulder with both hands as shown to stretch your lower back. Hold for 30 seconds. Relax. Repeat with the other leg.

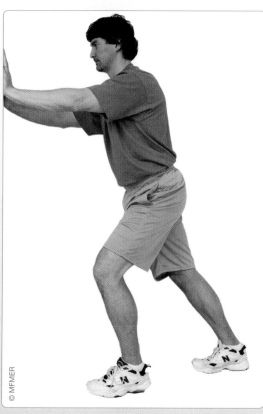

© MFMER

Calf stretch with straight knee

Stand an arm's length from the wall as shown. While maintaining a straight right knee (right heel on the floor), bend your left knee as if to move it toward the wall. This stretches your right calf. Hold for 30 seconds. Relax. Repeat with the other leg.

Benefits of stretching

Stretching is a powerful part of any exercise program. Regular stretching:

▶ Increases flexibility, which makes daily tasks easier and less tiring
▶ Improves range of motion in your joints, which keeps you mobile
▶ Improves circulation
▶ Promotes better posture
▶ Helps relieve stress by relaxing tense muscles
▶ Helps prevent injury, especially if your muscles or joints are tight

*If you have osteoporosis, avoid this stretch because it can increase the risk of a compression fracture in your spine.

Strengthening exercises

Strengthening exercises build stronger muscles to improve posture, balance and coordination. They also promote healthy bones, and they increase your rate of metabolism slightly, which can help keep your weight in check.

Here are four strengthening exercises. Start with about 15 repetitions of each. Use slow and controlled motions when lifting.

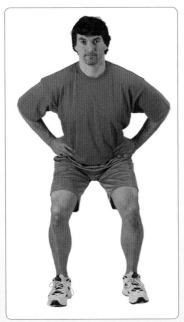

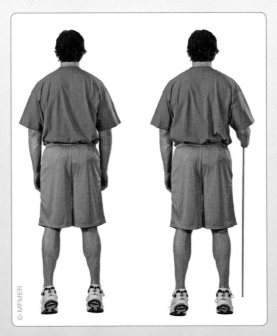

Wall or table pushups

Lean on a wall or table as shown. Slowly bend your elbows and lean your upper body toward the wall or table, supporting your weight with your arms and keeping your heels on the floor. Straighten your arms and return to the starting position.

Squat

To start, stand with your feet slightly more than shoulder-width apart. Put your hands on your waist or on a table or counter. Maintaining a normal back arch, slowly bend through the hips, knees and ankles as shown. Bend your knees as far as is comfortable, but no more than 90 degrees. Keep your knees in line with your feet and not ahead of your toes. Pause, then return to the starting position.

Calf strengthening

Stand with your feet shoulder-width apart. If necessary for balance, hold on to the back of a sturdy chair or another sturdy object. Slowly raise your heels from the floor and stand on your tiptoes. Hold. Slowly return to the starting position.

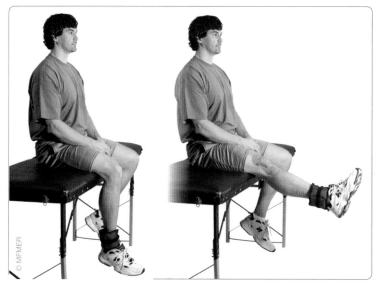

Knee extension*

Start as shown at left. Spine is in a neutral position. Maintaining alignment, slowly straighten your right knee as shown at right, pause, then return to the starting position. Do both legs.

*If you have a history of knee or back pain, avoid using an ankle weight until you improve your strength. People with back problems or older adults may want to use a chair with lumbar support.

Weight training: Do's and don'ts

In addition to strengthening exercises, there are many other ways to improve the strength of your muscles: resistance machines, resistance bands, free weights and other tools. Incorrect weight training technique is one of the main factors contributing to injuries. If you're just getting started, consider working with a weight training specialist. To stay safe and on track:

▶ **Set goals.** Make sure you and your trainer have a clear reason why you're doing each exercise and an overall goal for your program.
▶ **Lift an appropriate amount of weight.** If you're a beginner, you may be able to lift only 1 or 2 pounds — that's OK. Gradually work your way up.
▶ **Don't rush.** Don't jerk the weight up. Lift and lower the weight in a slow, smooth, controlled fashion.
▶ **Breathe.** Your blood pressure can increase to dangerous levels if you hold your breath during weight training. Exhale during the lift and essentially breathe freely during the process.
▶ **Seek balance.** Work all of your major muscles — abdominals, legs, chest, back, shoulders and arms.
▶ **Don't do too many sets of each exercise.** Completing one set of exercises to the point of fatigue is all you need to receive benefits.
▶ **Rest.** Give your body a day to recover between workouts of the same muscle group.
▶ **Be consistent.** Two workouts a week will build muscles, while one will maintain the strength you've gained.

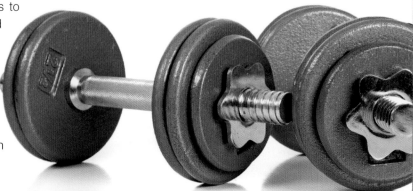

Use an activity log

Make copies of this log so that you have enough for the whole year. If you haven't been active, start slowly and build up your endurance. To continue improving, you may need to increase the amount of time you spend on fitness activities. Or you may find that you're exercising just the right amount to meet your goals.

Date	Activity	Category (aerobic, stretching, strengthening)	Amount of time

Avoiding injury

As you get more active, don't forget about safety. Follow these tips.

Wear proper clothing and shoes

Select clothes that are right for the weather and your activity. Physical activity increases your body temperature, so it's better to underdress than overdress. In cool weather, dress in layers so that you can remove or replace layers as you warm up or cool down.

In warm weather, wear lightweight, light-colored clothes. Sweating more won't help you lose fat, just water weight, which increases your risk of overheating and becoming dehydrated. Use sunscreen and wear a hat.

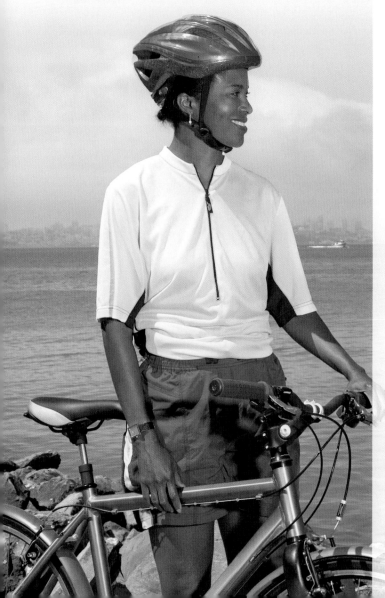

Make sure your shoes fit well and they aren't too tight. Replace them when they begin to show signs of wear. Always put on clean, smooth-fitting socks.

Examine your feet

Check your feet before you exercise. If you see any signs of irritation, cushion the area to avoid injury. If you have cuts, wash them with soap and water, use an antibiotic ointment, and bandage them.

After exercise, check your feet again. Look for blisters, warm areas or redness. If you have an open sore that doesn't heal, see a doctor.

Drink plenty of fluids

You lose fluid when you sweat, and it's important to replace this fluid. Water is the best choice. But if you're exercising for a long period, you may want the calories and electrolytes found in sports drinks. Drink fluids before, during and after exercise. The hotter the weather, the more important it is to keep your body hydrated.

Pay attention to your environment

Extreme temperatures can stress your body. On hot days, exercise indoors or early in the morning or late in the evening. In general, don't exercise outside if the temperature is higher than 80 F, especially if the humidity or the heat index is high. The heat index is based on a formula that uses both heat and humidity. Also avoid extremely cold temperatures.

Warm up and cool down

Before you begin exercising, get your body ready. Begin the exercise at a low intensity level and gradually increase the intensity level. For example, before you begin jogging or walking fast, walk for a few minutes at a slow or moderate pace to gradually increase your heart rate and oxygen flow in your lungs.

The same applies when you finish exercising — walk slowly for a while to allow your heart rate to gradually slow down. A couple of slow stretches afterward can help keep your muscles limber and prevent them from tightening up.

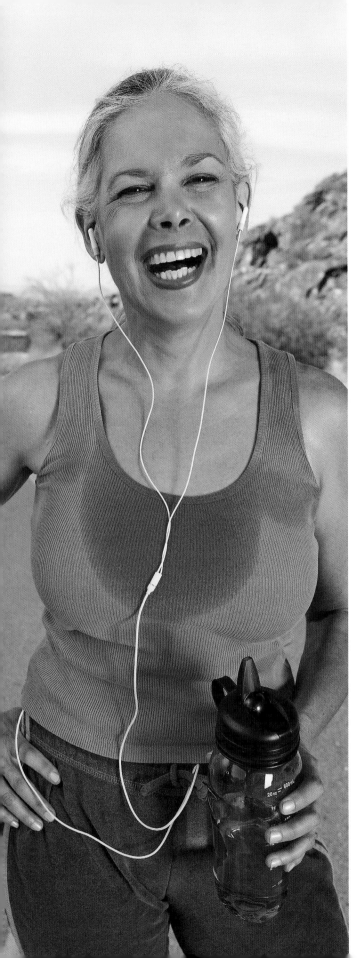

Exercise and regular monitoring

It's important that you track — monitor and record — your blood sugar (glucose) before, during and after exercise. This helps you and your health care team to learn how your body responds to exercise.

Exercise typically reduces your blood glucose level. During exercise, glucose that's stored in your muscles and liver is used for energy. After exercise, as your body rebuilds those stores, it takes glucose from your blood, lowering your blood glucose level.

Make sure that your blood glucose isn't too low before you begin exercising and that it doesn't drop too low during and after your workout. Blood glucose monitoring can also help prevent dangerous episodes of high blood glucose and high urine ketone levels.

Before exercise

To avoid swings in your blood glucose, test it about 30 minutes before you start and then once again immediately before exercising. This can help you determine if your blood glucose level is stable, rising or falling before you start to exercise.

The following blood glucose level guidelines can help you avoid problems during exercise:

- Less than 100 mg/dL. Eat a small carbohydrate-containing snack such as fruit or crackers. Test your glucose level after 15 to 30 minutes. Wait until your glucose level is at least 100 mg/dL before starting to exercise.
- 100 to 250 mg/dL. For most people, this is a safe pre-exercise blood glucose range.
- 250 mg/dL or higher. Before exercising, test your urine for ketones. If the results show a moderate or high level of ketones, don't exercise. Wait until your test indicates a low ketone level. Excess ketones indicate that your body doesn't have enough insulin to control your blood glucose, and this can lead to a life-threatening condition called diabetic ketoacidosis (DKA).
- 300 mg/dL or higher. Don't exercise. You need to bring your blood glucose down before you can

safely exercise because you risk an even greater increase in glucose. And high blood sugar (hyperglycemia) can lead to increased urination, which may result in dehydration.

During exercise

It's especially important to check your blood glucose during exercise if you're starting aerobic exercise for the first time, trying a new activity or sport, or increasing the intensity or duration of your workout.

If you exercise for more than an hour, especially if you have type 1 diabetes, stop and test your blood glucose every 30 minutes. Carry glucose sources with you to treat symptoms of low blood glucose. If your blood glucose is less than 100 mg/dL, or if it's not that low but you have symptoms of low blood glucose — feeling shaky, weak, anxious, sweaty or confused — eat a snack that serves as a fast-acting source of glucose. Examples include:

▶ A few glucose tablets
▶ ½ cup of fruit juice
▶ ½ cup of a regular (not diet) soft drink
▶ About five pieces of hard candy

Recheck your blood glucose 15 minutes after this snack. If it's still too low, have another serving and test yourself again 15 minutes later, until your glucose reaches 100 mg/dL or higher.

After exercise

The more strenuous the workout, the longer your blood glucose is affected. Check your blood glucose a couple of times after exercising to make sure you aren't developing hypoglycemia, which can occur even hours after you've stopped.

Be patient

You may think that testing your blood glucose before, during and after you exercise sounds like a lot of time and effort. But keep in mind that once you know how your body responds to exercise, you may not need to check your blood glucose as often — follow your doctor's advice.

Getting and staying motivated

Motivation is at the heart of your fitness plan — it's what gets you going and keeps you at it. By understanding what motivates you, you'll be better able to follow through with your fitness plan. For most people, getting started on a fitness program is the hardest step. But you can change the beliefs that keep you stuck.

Recognize what does or doesn't motivate you

Ask yourself what can you do differently to help you succeed this time.

Ask for support

Explain your fitness plans to your friends and family. Who can you exercise with, or who can support you in other ways?

Focus on the process and take small steps

Set realistic, attainable goals and continue to reassess them.

Monitor your progress

Keep track of your progress as you go along. Use a weekly activity log or a computer spreadsheet.

Tips for staying motivated

To get and stay motivated for the long haul:

▶ Make a commitment and don't look too far ahead. What can you do today to make this fitness plan work for you?
▶ Expand your definition of fitness activity. It's not just working out in the gym — it's any physical activity.
▶ Take that first step. You'll likely get motivated once you start. Even if it's a small step, get moving. Don't wait for motivation to come to you.
▶ Avoid all-or-nothing thinking. If you don't have time to do your usual routine, do less, but do something. The next day, try to do more.

Positive self-talk

Whenever you think about something, you are, in a sense, talking to yourself. Psychologists refer to this as self-talk. Becoming conscious of what you're saying to yourself and making it more positive can help you break bad habits, boost self-confidence and encourage you to stick with your exercise program.

Positive self-talk can increase your energy, motivation and positive attitude, while negative self-talk is critical and anxiety producing. Instructional self-talk helps you improve your performance by focusing on a technique or how to do something.

One proven technique for overcoming defeating self-talk is to replace negative thoughts with positive ones. Here are some examples, but remember it takes time and patience.

Negative self-talk	Positive self-talk
"I'm so tired."	"I'm going to feel more energized."
"I should be better at this by now."	"I've made some real improvements, and I'm where I need to be."
"Skipping this one walk won't matter."	"Every little bit makes a big difference."
"I'll never stick with this exercise program."	"Just take one day at a time and have fun."
"I'll never recover from this injury."	"Healing takes time. I'll just continue to do something every day."

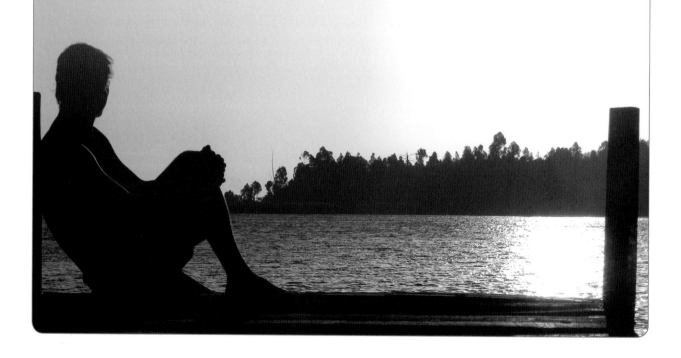

Have you hit a plateau?

You've been working out for a few months, and you're not seeing the same kind of results as you did in the beginning. What's going on?

You may have hit a plateau in your fitness program. This sense of running into a wall is familiar to many exercisers. Unless you update your program regularly, you'll likely come to a plateau at some point.

What you can do

After several weeks of working out at the same intensity and duration or lifting the same amount of weight with the same number of repetitions, your body adapts to that level of activity and you may not see the same results as you did in the beginning. This is known as a plateau. You won't see continued improvements unless you alter your routine.

You may need to increase the frequency, duration or intensity of your activities. Varying your activities also may help you avoid plateaus, as can switching the order in which you do your exercises. Sometimes you reach a plateau when you're bored, you lose interest in your activity, or you're tired of the same routine.

A plateau doesn't have to be a pitfall. If you find yourself stalling out, take action. First figure out the cause of the plateau and then determine an appropriate solution.

When's the best time to exercise?

The best time to exercise depends on your diabetes treatment. If you take insulin, avoid exercising for the three hours after injecting rapid- or short-acting insulin because of the potential risk of low blood sugar (glucose). Both insulin and exercise lower your blood glucose. Ask your doctor whether you need to adjust your insulin dose before exercising and how long you should wait to exercise after injecting insulin.

Don't exercise for more than an hour unless you've discussed your insulin needs with your doctor. If you have type 1 diabetes and you exercise for more than an hour or do strenuous activities, you may benefit from a snack before you begin or while exercising.

For most people with type 2 diabetes, a snack before exercise generally isn't necessary. If you don't take medications to control your diabetes, it also may be OK to exercise after you eat, when your blood glucose level is generally highest.

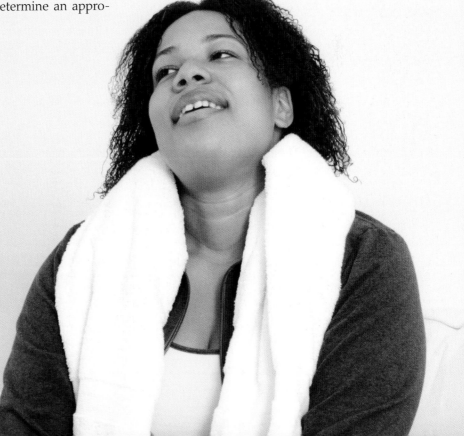

Fitness for kids

To keep your kids healthy, it's important to get them off the couch! Use these tips to help your kids develop a lifelong appreciation for activities that increase their fitness.

▶ **Set a good example.** If you want active kids, be active yourself. Talk about physical activity as an opportunity to take care of your body, rather than a punishment or a chore.

▶ **Limit screen time.** Consider limiting screen time — TV, video games and computer time — to two hours a day. Don't put a TV in your children's bedrooms, and keep the computer in a family area. Limit other sedentary activities, such as chatting on the phone.

▶ **Choose video games that require movement.** Activity-oriented video games — dance games and video games that use physical movements to control screen action — boost calorie-burning power. In a Mayo Clinic study, kids who traded sedentary screen time for active screen time more than doubled their energy expenditure.

▶ **Establish a routine.** Set aside time each day for physical activity. Get up early with your children to walk the dog or do jumping jacks together after dinner. Gradually add new activities to the routine as you all become more fit.

▶ **Encourage your children to walk to school** (if feasible). If school is within walking distance, encourage your older kids to walk. For younger children, talk with parents and others in the neighborhood to see if you can rotate responsibility for walking the neighborhood kids to school.

▶ **Let your children set the pace.** Organized sports are a great way to stay fit, but they aren't for everyone. What interests your child? If it's reading, walk or bike to the neighborhood library. If it's art, take a nature hike to collect leaves and make a picture. If it's music, dance to your child's favorite music.

Keep it fun

To keep your kids interested in fitness, make it fun for them:

▶ **Be silly.** Let younger children see how much fun you can have while being active. Run like a gorilla. Walk like a spider. Hop like a bunny.

▶ **Get in the game.** Play catch, get the whole family involved in a game of tag or have a jump-rope contest.

▶ **Make chores a friendly challenge.** Who can pull the most weeds out of the garden? Who can collect the most litter in the neighborhood?

▶ **Try an activity party.** For your child's next birthday, schedule a bowling party, take the kids to a climbing wall or set up relay races in the backyard.

▶ **Put your kids in charge.** Let each child take a turn choosing the activity of the day or week. The key is to find things that your children like to do.

Make it an escape

If you prefer to get your exercise away from home, here are some suggestions:

▶ **Get social.** Your children may do better with the encouragement of others. Consider signing them up for a dance club, hiking group or golf league.

▶ **Join a team.** Sign up for a softball, soccer or volleyball team through your company or through your local parks and recreation department. A team commitment is a great motivator.

▶ **Join a fitness club.** Sign up for a group exercise class at a nearby fitness club. The money you're paying out each month may be an incentive to stick with it.

▶ **Plan active outings.** Make a date with a friend to hike in a local park or take a family trip to the zoo.

▶ **Stay active during errands.** When shopping, park at the back of the lot and walk farther to your destination.

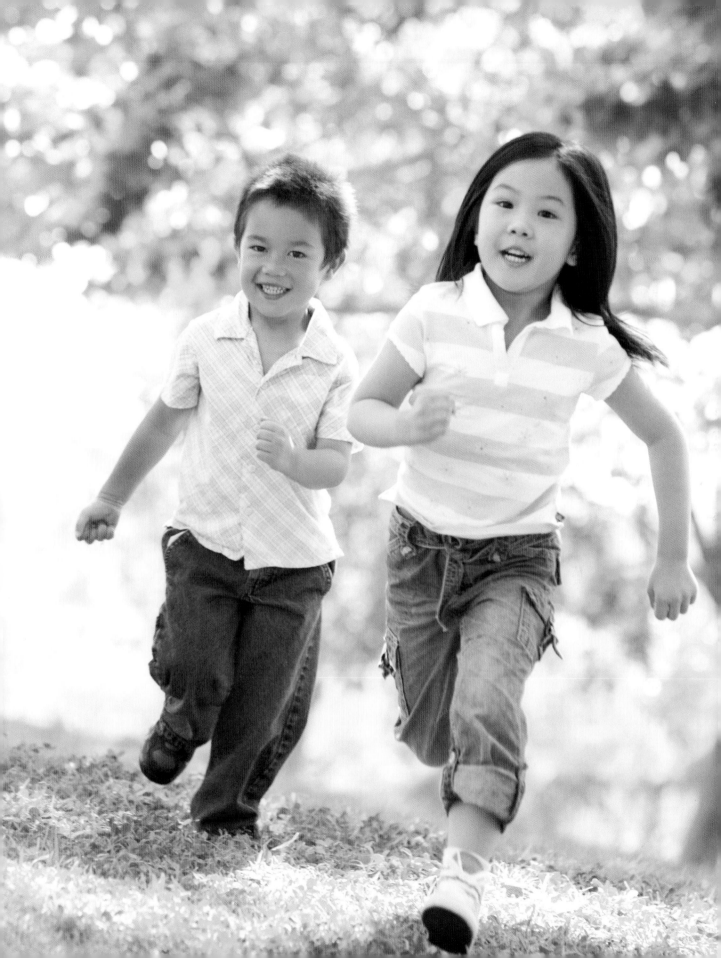

Chapter 6
Medical Treatment

Insulin therapy 144

How to inject insulin 149

Avoiding insulin problems 153

Insulin pumps 154

Oral diabetes medications 156

Oral drug combinations 162

Oral drugs and insulin 162

Injectable drugs 164

Kidney dialysis 165

Kidney transplant 167

Other transplant procedures 167

A visit with Dr. Pankaj Shah

"If managing your diabetes seems overwhelming, take it one day at a time. And remember that you're not in it alone. Working as a team with your doctor and a diabetes educator, you can control your diabetes and prevent its complications — and do it with minimal disruption of your regular lifestyle."

Now that you've been diagnosed with diabetes, it's very important that you work closely with your doctor to define the goals of your treatment and the best strategy to meet those goals. Maintaining good control of your blood sugar (glucose) is very important, as it's been shown that good control is key to preventing many of the long-term complications of poorly controlled diabetes, such as eye problems (diabetic retinopathy, which can lead to blindness), loss of kidney function and eventual need for dialysis, and nerve damage (neuropathy) that can result in loss of sensation or pain in the feet, foot ulcers, and, in some cases, amputation. All of these problems are preventable. If you already have any of them, controlling your blood sugar can delay their progression to a more severe or advanced state.

A healthy diet and regular exercise to maintain a healthy weight are an essential part of diabetes treatment, and for many people with type 2 diabetes, they may be the only measures needed — at least early in the course of the disease. When diet and exercise aren't sufficient to maintain acceptable blood sugar levels, your doctor may prescribe oral medications or sometimes injectable medications, including insulin. Many times, in order to maintain good blood sugar control, people need a combination of oral medications that affect blood sugar in different ways or a combination of oral drugs and injectable medications, such as insulin.

The purpose of medication is to keep your blood sugar level as close to normal as possible to delay or prevent complications. Tight control of blood sugar levels can reduce the risk of diabetes-related complications, including heart attack, stroke, and nerve, kidney and eye problems, by more than 50 percent.

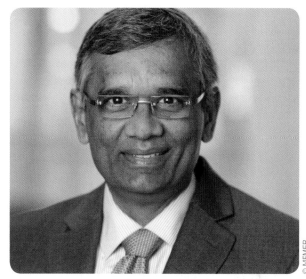

Pankaj Shah, M.D.
Endocrinology

For people with type 1 diabetes, insulin injections are necessary. You may need to take insulin injections several times a day, and the amount of insulin needed will depend on your blood sugar levels and the foods you eat. At some point, your doctor may recommend an insulin pump. You'll need to work closely with your doctor and your diabetes educator to determine whether the dose of insulin you're taking is appropriate or whether it needs to be adjusted. Periodic follow-up with your doctor and a diabetes educator to determine the adequacy of your treatment is important.

With both type 1 and type 2 diabetes, your doctor will likely perform certain tests to help him or her decide if your medication needs to be adjusted, and also to determine if there's any evidence that complications may be developing so that they can be treated in a timely manner.

If managing your diabetes seems overwhelming, take it one day at a time. And remember that you're not in it alone. Working as a team with your doctor and a diabetes educator, you can control your diabetes and prevent its complications — and do it all with minimal disruption of your regular lifestyle.

If you have diabetes, there are several approaches to help manage your blood sugar (glucose). Many people with type 2 diabetes are able to control their disease with proper eating and exercise and by maintaining a healthy weight.

However, for some people, lifestyle changes alone aren't enough. They need medication to keep their blood glucose within a healthy range.

For individuals with type 1 diabetes, insulin is a must. Insulin injections are necessary to replace the insulin the pancreas no longer produces.

Insulin therapy

Treatment with insulin, called insulin therapy, has two goals:

▶ To maintain blood glucose at near-normal levels or within the target range that your doctor recommends
▶ To prevent long-term complications of diabetes

The most widely used insulins are slight modifications of the "human" insulin. These are manufactured in a laboratory. Some insulins, known as insulin analogs, are modified by the manufacturer to better mimic normal insulin secretion by the pancreas.

Your doctor will decide which insulin treament is best for you. That will depend on:

When insulin isn't enough

A few years ago, the Food and Drug Administration approved use of a medication to help treat type 1 diabetes called pramlintide (Symlin).

Pramlintide is only for adults with type 1 or type 2 diabetes who use insulin and need better control of their blood sugar (glucose).

Taken as an injection before you eat, pramlintide can help lower blood glucose during the three hours after meals. For more information on this drug, see page 164.

▶ Trends and patterns of your blood glucose levels
▶ Your lifestyle
▶ What you eat
▶ How much you exercise
▶ Whether you have other health conditions

Types of insulin

Many types of insulin are available. They differ in the time it takes the drug to begin working (onset), at what point the insulin has the most effect (peak) and how long the overall effect lasts (duration).

Insulin is administered by an injection or through continuous infusion from an insulin pump. You and your health care team will determine the type and amount of insulin that best meets your needs. See the chart on pages 146 and 147.

Pre-mixed insulin

Pre-mixed insulin combines rapid- or short-acting insulin with intermediate-acting insulin. This is convenient if you need two types of insulin but have trouble drawing up insulin out of two bottles, or you have poor eyesight or have arthritis or other problems with your hands.

There are several pre-mixed insulins, and some have long generic names. The numbers after each brand name show that the bottle contains two types of insulin in different percentages (such as 70 percent intermediate-acting insulin and 30 percent short-acting insulin):

▶ Humulin 70/30
▶ Novolin 70/30
▶ NovoLog Mix 70/30
▶ Humalog Mix 75/25
▶ Novolin/ReliOn 70/30

Because you're getting two types of insulin, the onset, peak and duration of each type will differ but overlap. Follow the directions of your doctor or diabetes educator. Typically if the pre-mixed product has short-acting insulin, you'll inject it 30 minutes before a meal; if the product has rapid-acting insulin, you'll inject it no more than 15 minutes before your meal.

Insulin regimens

There are several types of insulin dosage options.

Single dose

You inject a dose of intermediate-acting or long-acting insulin once each day.

Mixed dose

You inject rapid- or short-acting insulin and intermediate-acting insulin — mixed in one syringe.

Pre-mixed dose

You inject a dose of pre-mixed insulin once or twice a day.

Split dose

You give yourself two injections of intermediate-acting insulin each day. These injections are usually given before breakfast and before the evening meal, or before breakfast and at bedtime.

Split mixed dose

You give yourself two injections that contain a combination of a rapid- or short-acting insulin and an intermediate-acting insulin — mixed in one syringe — each day. These are generally given before breakfast and before the evening meal.

Split pre-mixed dose

You give yourself two injections of pre-mixed insulin daily. They're usually given before breakfast and before the evening meal.

Intensive therapy

This regimen involves multiple daily injections of insulin or using a small portable pump that continuously administers insulin.

Intensive insulin therapy

People taking insulin have less risk of complications from their diabetes if they can keep their blood glucose as near to normal as safely possible.

For people with type 1 diabetes, the preferred therapy used to achieve this is intensive insulin therapy. People with type 2 diabetes also can benefit from intensive insulin therapy if medications and lifestyle changes don't keep blood glucose levels in the target range.

Intensive insulin therapy involves monitoring your blood glucose frequently, using a combination of insulins, and adjusting your insulin doses based on your blood glucose levels, diet and changes in your routine. When practiced effectively, intensive insulin therapy can greatly lower complication risks.

If your doctor recommends intensive insulin therapy, there are two options:

Multiple daily injections

You take three or more injections of insulin each day — often a combination of types — to achieve tight control of your blood glucose.

Insulin pump

An insulin pump continuously releases rapid- or short-acting insulin into your body through a plastic tube placed underneath the skin on your abdomen (see page 154).

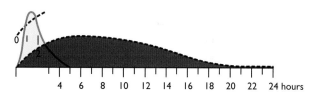

Comparing rapid- and intermediate-acting insulins
This shows an example of the difference between rapid-acting (solid line) and intermediate-acting (broken line) insulins in time of onset, peak and duration.

© MFMER

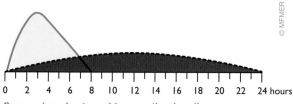

Comparing short- and long-acting insulins
This shows an example of the difference between short-acting (solid line) and long-acting (broken line) insulins in time of onset, peak and duration.

Insulin options

You and your health care team will determine the type and amount of insulin that best meets your needs. Below are examples, but talk with your doctor and check the package insert of the product for complete information. Keep in mind that:

▶ Onset of action means how soon the insulin starts to lower blood glucose
▶ Peak action means when the insulin works the strongest
▶ Duration means how long the overall effect lasts

Type of insulin	Insulin name (brand name)	Onset of action
Rapid-acting insulin Absorbed more quickly than short-acting insulin and effects wear off sooner	Insulin aspart (NovoLog) Insulin glulisine (Apidra) Insulin lispro (Humalog)	5 to 15 minutes
Short-acting insulin Works quickly, but effects don't last as long as intermediate-acting insulin	Insulin regular (Humulin R, Novolin R, Novolin/ReliOn R)	30 to 60 minutes
Intermediate-acting insulin Starts working later than short-acting insulin and effects last longer	neutral protamine Hagedorn, or NPH (Humulin N, Novolin N, Novolin/ReliOn N)	1 to 2 hours
Long-acting insulin Takes several hours to work, but provides insulin at a steady level for up to 24 hours	Insulin glargine (Lantus) Insulin detemir (Levemir)	1 to 2 hours 2 hours

*Follow the advice of your doctor. Onset, peak and duration times are estimates — times vary among individuals and are affected by the site of injection and other issues, such as when you last ate or exercised.
Product manufacturers and the American Diabetes Association, 2012

Peak action	Duration	How it's typically used*
30 minutes to 2 hours (range varies by product)	3 to 4 hours (range varies by product)	Inject immediately before a meal — can cause blood glucose to drop too low (hypoglycemia) if injected too early before a meal. Often used in addition to intermediate- or long-acting insulin. Commonly used in insulin pumps.
2 to 4 hours (range varies by product)	6 to 8 hours (range varies by product)	Inject 30 minutes before a meal. May be used in addition to intermediate- or long-acting insulin.
4 to 12 hours (range varies by product)	16 to 24 hours (range varies by product)	Generally covers insulin needs for about half a day. Should last overnight when used just before bedtime. May be used in addition to rapid- or short-acting insulin. Should not be used with insulin pumps.
No clear peak	Up to 24 hours	Effects last for about a day. Should not be mixed with other types of insulin in one syringe but may be used in addition to rapid- or short-acting insulin. Should not be used in insulin pumps.
No clear peak	14 to 16 hours	

Drawbacks of intensive insulin therapy

Intensive insulin therapy has two possible drawbacks: low blood glucose (hypoglycemia) and weight gain.

When your blood glucose is already close to normal, hypoglycemia can occur even with minor changes in your routine, such as an unexpected increase in activity. You can counter this risk by being aware of changes in your routine that increase your risk of hypoglycemia.

It's also important to recognize the signs and symptoms of low blood glucose and respond quickly when you begin to experience them (see page 22).

Weight gain can occur because when you use more insulin to control your blood glucose, more glucose gets into your cells and less glucose is wasted in your urine. Glucose that's not used by your cells accumulates as fat.

Work with your team

Talk with your doctor to find out if intensive insulin therapy is for you. You'll likely need to measure your blood glucose level more often, and if you take insulin, you may need to change your dosing schedule. But remember that healthy eating and exercising also are vital for glucose control. Think of these actions as key factors that can add years to your life.

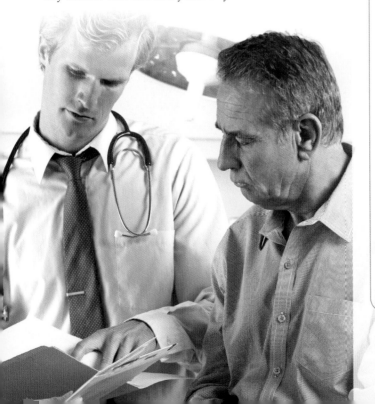

Tight glucose control: Preventing complications

Several studies confirm that tight blood sugar (glucose) control — keeping your blood glucose as near normal as safely possible — can dramatically reduce your risk of developing complications.

Diabetes Control and Complications Trial

In the 10-year Diabetes Control and Complications Trial (DCCT), more than 1,400 volunteers with type 1 diabetes were randomly assigned to one of two groups:

1. The conventional group received the routine insulin therapy recommended by their doctors.
2. The intensive therapy group received intensive insulin therapy using multiple daily injections or an insulin pump.

The goal was to keep the trial participants' blood glucose as close to normal as possible. Results showed that tight blood glucose control using intensive insulin therapy reduced the risk of many complications — such as eye damage or kidney disease — by at least 50 percent compared with those receiving conventional treatment.

United Kingdom Prospective Diabetes Study

The United Kingdom Prospective Diabetes Study (UKPDS) recruited more than 5,100 people with newly diagnosed type 2 diabetes. Participants were followed for an average of 10 years. Overall, the results showed that people who tried to keep their blood glucose at a normal level had one-fourth fewer complications involving their eyes, kidneys and nerves. Improved blood glucose and blood pressure control also led to a reduced risk of heart disease. Benefits of good glucose control were observed even a decade or more after the studies were completed.

How to inject insulin

When you first learn that you need to take insulin, you may feel frightened or nervous about injecting yourself with the medication. That's natural. Learning about the process and doing it a few times will help you feel more comfortable.

The most common way to receive insulin is by syringe — either one that you fill yourself or a pre-filled syringe. This method delivers insulin underneath the skin, where it's absorbed into the bloodstream.

Selecting a site

Insulin may be injected into any area of your body where a layer of fatty tissue is present and where large blood vessels, nerves, muscles and bones aren't close to the surface.

Insulin is best injected into the abdomen because this location allows for quick and consistent absorption. However, avoid the 2-inch radius around the navel, which doesn't absorb as well. Rotate the injection site to avoid or reduce indentations, thickened skin or hard lumps from the injections.

If appropriate, your doctor or diabetes educator may recommend alternative areas for injection, such as your upper arms, thighs or buttocks.

After you determine the site for your insulin injection, it's recommended to clean the site with an alcohol wipe or soap and water. After you've cleaned the site, be sure to allow it to dry before giving yourself an injection.

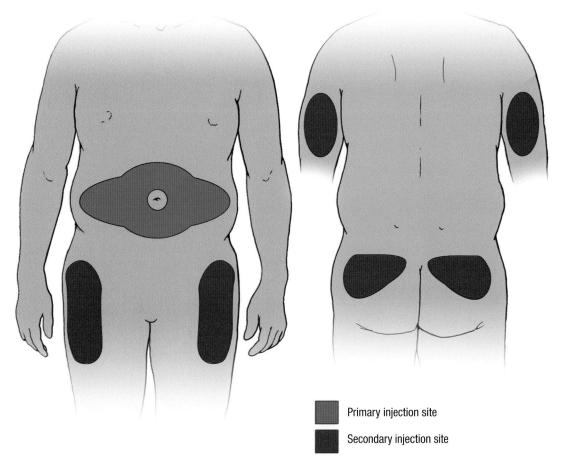

■ Primary injection site

■ Secondary injection site

© MFMER

Generally the abdomen is the best injection site. Rotate the site of each injection within the abdomen. The thighs and upper arms (shaded areas) as well as the buttocks also are potential injection sites.

Drawing insulin into a syringe

With time and practice, the process of drawing insulin into a syringe becomes routine and is no longer so daunting. Here's how to do it:

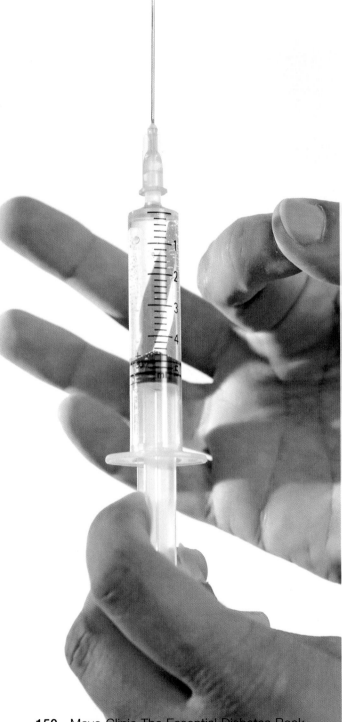

▶ Gather your supplies: bottle of insulin, syringe and needle, alcohol wipe, and a covered, puncture-resistant container for needle discard.

▶ Check the label on the insulin bottle for the type, concentration and expiration date. Use the same type of insulin every time, unless your doctor tells you otherwise. Changing insulin types may affect blood glucose control.

▶ Check the insulin bottle for any changes in the insulin. Make sure no clumping, frosting, precipitation, or change in clarity or color has occurred, which may mean that the insulin has lost potency.

▶ Wash your hands with soap and water.

▶ Clear insulin doesn't need to be mixed. However, cloudy insulin should be mixed by gently rolling the bottle between your hands. (Don't shake the bottle — that may decrease the insulin's potency.) Then, check to make sure there are no particles at the bottom of the bottle.

▶ Wipe off the top of the insulin bottle with an alcohol wipe.

▶ Remove the needle cap from the sterile syringe.

▶ Pull the plunger to draw in an amount of air equal to the amount of insulin that you need.

▶ Insert the needle through the rubber stopper of the insulin bottle, and push the plunger so that air goes into the bottle. This equalizes air pressure in the bottle, making it easier to withdraw the insulin.

▶ While keeping the needle in the bottle, turn the bottle upside down.

▶ Pull the plunger on the syringe and withdraw insulin, not air, slightly past the number of units needed. Air isn't dangerous, but it reduces the amount of insulin in the syringe.

▶ If there are air bubbles, remove them. Either push the insulin back into the bottle (without taking the needle out of the bottle) and draw it again, or snap the syringe sharply with your finger and then push the plunger to expel the air into the bottle.

▶ Recheck the syringe for air. If air is present, repeat the previous step.

▶ Double-check the amount of insulin in the syringe.

▶ Pull the needle out of the bottle.

It may seem like a lot of steps to prepare for the injection, but once you become comfortable with injecting yourself, it takes very little time.

Injecting the insulin

Once you have the right amount of insulin in the syringe and you've removed the needle from the bottle, it's time to inject the insulin. To do so effectively:

▶ **Hold the syringe like a pencil.** Quickly insert the entire length of the needle into a pinched fold of your skin at a 90-degree angle. (If you're thin, you may need to use a short needle or inject at a 45-degree angle to avoid injecting into your muscle, especially in the thigh area.)

▶ **Release the pinched skin.** Inject the insulin by gently pushing the syringe's plunger all the way down at a steady, moderate rate. Pause for five seconds, then withdraw the needle from your skin at the same angle it went in. (If the plunger jams as you're injecting the insulin, remove the needle and note the number of units remaining in the syringe. Contact your doctor or diabetes educator for advice.)

▶ **Don't re-cap the needle.** Discard it in a covered, puncture-resistant container.

Avoid injection site problems

Occasionally — especially when you first start using insulin — you may notice redness and slight swelling at the injection site. It could be the result of impurities in the insulin, or it could stem from a small amount of alcohol getting into fat tissues.

To avoid this, let the injection site dry after cleaning it with alcohol. If the skin irritation lasts more than two to three weeks or causes you discomfort, talk with your doctor.

To reduce painful injections:

▶ Make sure the insulin is at room temperature.
▶ Be sure no air bubbles are in the syringe.
▶ Relax your muscles in the area of the injection.
▶ Penetrate your skin quickly with the needle.
▶ Don't change the direction of the needle.

Some people develop indentations, hard lumps or thickened skin in areas where they inject insulin. Try to avoid injecting in these areas because the insulin won't be absorbed well. Rotating the site of your injections may prevent or reduce this problem.

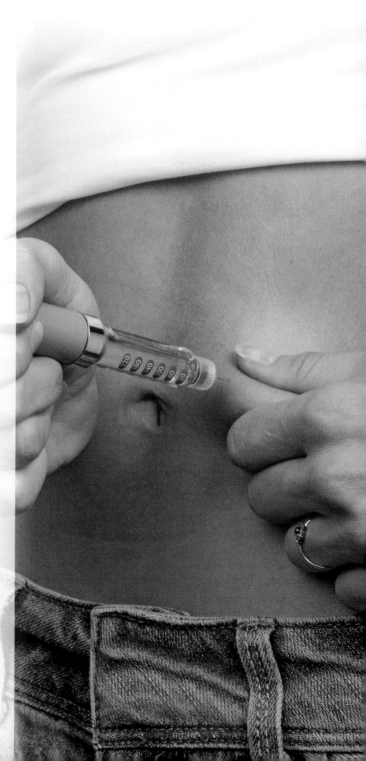

Alternatives to a syringe and needle

The insulin pen and insulin jet injector are options to the syringe and needle for insulin delivery. An insulin pump (see page 154) is another alternative. All of these options have their pros and cons. Discuss alternative devices with your doctor to determine which method is best for you. And find out what your insurance covers before you buy.

Insulin pen

This device looks like a pen with a cartridge (as shown below). Refillable pens have pre-filled disposable cartridges that contain insulin. Other pens are completely disposable. You place a fine-point needle, much like the one on a syringe, on the tip of the pen. You turn a dial to select the desired insulin dose, insert the needle under your skin and click down on a button at the end of the pen to deliver the insulin. If you have arthritis, a disposable insulin pen is convenient because you won't have to load and unload insulin cartridges.

A disposable insulin pen with large numbers on the dial may work best if you have vision problems.

Insulin jet injector

This device uses high-pressure air to send a fine spray of insulin under your skin. There may be some discomfort and possible bruising. This device may not be as accurate as other methods because some of the insulin can be lost during injection. Jet injectors are more expensive than are pen injectors.

Future of insulin delivery

Researchers continue to explore new methods of insulin delivery, such as patches, pills, an oral spray and the "artificial pancreas"— an integrated insulin delivery system, consisting of an insulin pump, a glucose sensor and a third device, usually a smartphone or an equivalent device that integrates the information from the sensor with factors such as your activity and food intake in order to determine the amount of insulin to be delivered.

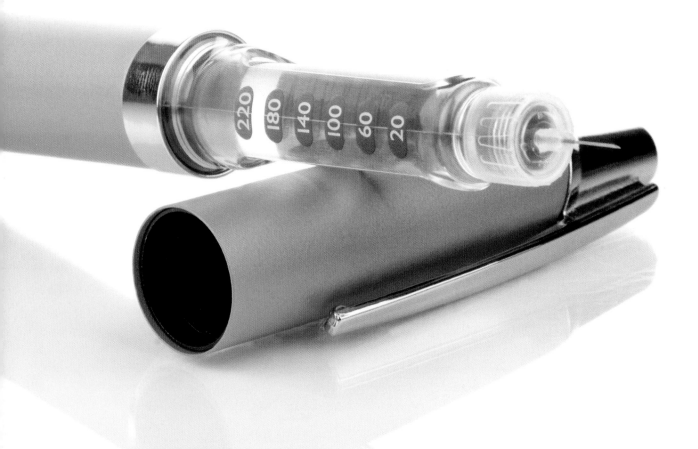

Avoiding insulin problems

The following steps can reduce your risk of problems from insulin use.

Buy all of your insulin from the same pharmacy
This will help ensure that you receive the type and concentration of insulin that's prescribed and alert you to changes in your prescription. Check the expiration date on the package and always keep a spare bottle on hand.

Speak up
To avoid possible drug interactions or drug side effects, inform your pharmacist, dentist and those health professionals who may not be familiar with your medical history that you take insulin.

Store your insulin in the refrigerator until it's opened
After a bottle has been opened, it may be kept at room temperature for one month. Insulin at room temperature causes less discomfort when injected. Throw away your insulin after the expiration date or after it's been kept at room temperature for a month.

Avoid temperature extremes
Never freeze insulin or expose it to extremely hot temperatures or direct sunlight.

Look for changes in appearance
Throw away insulin that's discolored or contains solid particles.

Wear diabetes identification
Wear an identification necklace or bracelet that identifies you as an insulin user. In addition, carry an identification card that includes the name and phone number of your doctor and all the medications you're taking, including the kind of insulin. In case your blood glucose drops too low, this will help people know how to respond.

Check all medications
Before taking any medication other than your insulin, including over-the-counter products, read the warning label. If the label says you shouldn't take the drug if you have diabetes, consult your doctor before taking it.

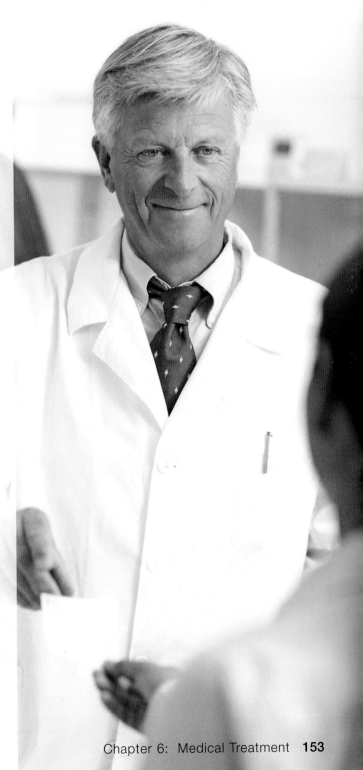

Insulin pumps

An insulin pump is a computerized device that's about the size of a pager or small cellphone. Some pumps are worn on your belt or in your pocket, while others stick to your skin. The pump provides a continuous supply of insulin, eliminating the need for daily shots.

The pump has a container that you fill with insulin. A small, flexible tube connects the container of insulin to a catheter that's inserted under the skin of your abdomen. You use a needle to insert the catheter and then withdraw the needle.

Based on information that you program into the device, the pump delivers a continuous (basal) infusion of short- or rapid-acting insulin and extra insulin (bolus) before meals to cover an expected rise in blood glucose from the meals.

Every second or third day you need to change the infusion site. To do this, you pull out the catheter and insert a new one at a different site. Your doctor or diabetes educator will likely recommend that you rotate the injection site among the four quadrants of your abdomen. The reservoir that holds the insulin also needs to be refilled every few days.

If you decide to use an insulin pump, you'll typically go through thorough training in all aspects of pump use. During this training you'll learn how to determine your insulin requirements, how to program your pump to safely administer the insulin, and how to insert the catheter and care for the injection site.

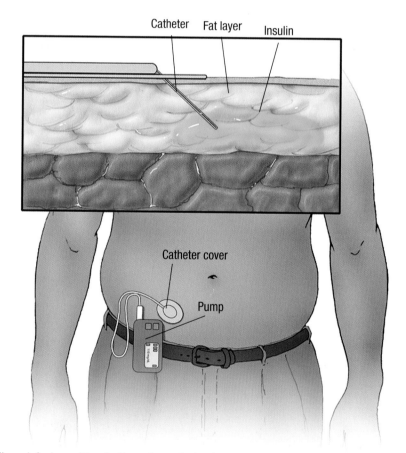

An insulin pump delivers infusions of insulin through a catheter that's placed in the layer of fat under the skin on your abdomen. The pump is programmed to dispense specific amounts of insulin automatically. It can be programmed to deliver more or less insulin depending on your meals, activity level and blood sugar level.

Convenience and control

Several studies have confirmed the effectiveness of insulin pump therapy, known as continuous sub-cutaneous insulin infusion (CSII). The main advantage of an insulin pump is convenience. It may also improve glucose control and reduce the risks of low blood glucose.

Most people who use an insulin pump feel that the pump allows a more flexible lifestyle. Other advantages include:

- Built-in safety alarms to let you know if the line's plugged, you're out of insulin or the battery is low
- Memory display of previous insulin delivery
- The ability to program different rates of insulin delivery to help prevent low and high blood sugar levels
- The ability to control meal-related insulin delivery
- The ability to suspend or decrease insulin delivery during physical activity
- Quick-release technology to easily disconnect the infusion tubing for situations such as showering, swimming or engaging in sexual activity
- Better blood glucose control in hard-to-control situations, such as travel, variable work shifts and erratic schedules

Who's a candidate?

Insulin pumps can be beneficial, but they aren't for everybody. If you're doing a good job of controlling your diabetes without a pump, the investment may not bring significant improvements.

To benefit from a pump you need to use it properly, monitor your blood glucose regularly, and work closely with your doctor and diabetes educator. Some people find this too demanding.

The pumps also are expensive, costing up to several thousand dollars. However, this cost is covered, in full or in part, by insurance.

Other drawbacks include risk of infection at the pump site, high blood glucose if the pump fails to deliver insulin and difficulty incorporating the pump into some physical activities.

Some women with diabetes who are pregnant or are trying to become pregnant prefer an insulin pump. High blood glucose in early pregnancy can cause birth defects and illness in infants. Tight blood glucose control reduces that risk.

There are several other situations for which an insulin pump may be beneficial.

Episodes of severe low blood glucose
An insulin pump can reduce the incidence of severe hypoglycemia.

Poor control despite multiple injection therapy
Insulin pump therapy can match the insulin needs of some people better than can insulin injections.

Extreme insulin sensitivity
A pump can deliver very small amounts of insulin, which is hard to do with injections.

Dawn effect
Some people experience increased glucose production in the early morning hours, called the dawn effect, and need more insulin at that time. A pump can increase insulin delivery during that time.

Variable schedules
A pump allows you the freedom to program your insulin doses to meet your changing needs.

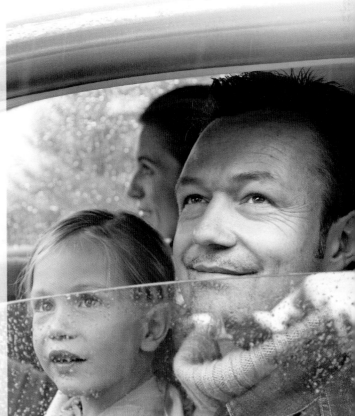

Using the pump correctly

People who use a pump can't be afraid of mechanical devices. And it's essential that you have a clear understanding of the relationship between insulin, food and activity so that you can program your pump to help you in changing situations.

Even when using a insulin pump, you will still need to check your blood glucose several times a day. It's also important to meet regularly with your doctor or diabetes educator to make sure you're using the device correctly.

Oral diabetes medications

If you have type 2 diabetes, there are several approaches to help manage your blood sugar (glucose). Although many people can control type 2 diabetes by eating properly, exercising and maintaining a healthy weight, lifestyle changes alone aren't enough for some people.

Your doctor may recommend medications to help control your blood glucose — but even so, remember that a healthy diet and regular exercise still play a key role.

Several classes of oral drugs are available. Each class has a different chemical structure and its own method for lowering blood glucose. Some oral medications stimulate your pancreas to release more insulin. Others make your body's cells more sensitive to the effects of insulin, and still others slow your body's absorption of carbohydrates.

Your doctor may recommend more than one drug, or you may need to take drugs along with insulin. Most people begin with an oral drug.

Talk with your doctor or a diabetes educator about the pros and cons of each drug — he or she will recommend an option based on your specific needs. The chart on pages 158 and 159 lists several classes of diabetes drugs, with examples of their main advantages and disadvantages.

The decision on which type of medication may be best for you is based on several factors, such as:

Implantable insulin pumps

An implantable insulin pump system is being clinically evaluated but is not yet available for public use in the United States. Implanting an insulin pump in your lower abdomen may be more convenient and less noticeable. The pump delivers small amounts of insulin throughout the day, which may help people who have a difficult time maintaining good glucose control.

▶ Whether you're overweight (some diabetes drugs cause weight gain)
▶ Your blood glucose levels and when they tend to rise (after meals, for example)
▶ Whether you have additional health problems
▶ Strength (potency) of the drug
▶ Possible side effects
▶ Cost, especially when several medications are needed to get your blood glucose under control

Sulfonylureas

Sulfonylureas (sul-fuh-nil-yoo-REE-uhs) have been used for decades to control blood glucose. The drugs work by stimulating beta cells in your pancreas to produce more insulin. So, to benefit from the medication, your pancreas must be able to produce some insulin on its own.

Glimepiride (Amaryl), glipizide (Glucotrol) and glyburide (DiaBeta, Glynase) are the most commonly used sulfonylureas. Glipizide is available in two forms: a short-acting version and a extended-release (XL) version.

Possible side effects

Low blood glucose (hypoglycemia) is a common side effect of sulfonylureas. You're at a much greater risk of developing hypoglycemia if you have impaired liver or kidney (renal) function. If you have one of these conditions, your doctor may decide not to prescribe a sulfonylurea and can recommend a different medication instead.

Precautions

Doing anything that reduces your blood glucose after you've taken a sulfonylurea, such as skipping a meal or exercising more than usual, can lead to low blood glucose. Taking alcohol or certain drugs with sulfonylureas, including decongestants, also can cause low blood glucose by boosting the effects of the medication. Medications such as steroids can decrease the effectiveness of sulfonylureas.

Biguanides

Biguanides (bi-GWAH-nides) improve your body's response to insulin, decreasing insulin resistance. Between meals your liver releases stored glucose into your bloodstream. Often too much glucose is released in people with type 2 diabetes. Biguanides reduce the amount of glucose your liver releases during fasting. As a result, you need less insulin to transport glucose from your blood to your individual cells.

Metformin (Glucophage) is the only drug in this class available in the United States. Metformin is also available in extended-release pills (Fortamet, Glucophage XR) and in liquid form (Riomet).

An important benefit of the drug is that it's associated with less weight gain than are other diabetes medications, and it may even promote weight loss. For this reason, it's often prescribed to overweight or obese people with type 2 diabetes. In addition, the drug may reduce blood fats (cholesterol and triglycerides), which tend to be higher than normal in people with type 2 diabetes.

Possible side effects

Metformin is generally well-tolerated, but it can produce side effects. These effects usually occur during the first few weeks and decrease with time. Often, lowering the dose or using the extended-release preparation would reduce these side effects.

Let your doctor know if you experience any of these side effects:

- Loss of appetite
- Nausea or vomiting
- Gas or diarrhea
- Abdominal bloating, discomfort or pain
- Changes in taste, such as an unpleasant metallic taste in your mouth

Precautions

Because of the increased risk of lactic acidosis, metformin usually isn't prescribed if you have kidney failure, liver failure, serious lung disease, heart failure or any other disease that may cause your body to produce too much lactic acid.

The following precautions also are important if you take this drug:

- If you drink alcohol daily or you occasionally overindulge, metformin and alcohol can produce lactic acidosis, making you sick. If you drink alcohol, discuss this with your doctor.
- Because of the potential for lactic acidosis, it's important to stop taking metformin before having any procedure that involves the use of an intravenous (IV) dye. IV dyes are sometimes used in imaging procedures, such as a computerized tomography (CT) scan.

? Are there any herbal remedies that will help treat type 2 diabetes?

Some people with diabetes do take herbal remedies in an effort to ease their symptoms, even though the effectiveness and side effects of these remedies are generally unknown. This is risky — manufacturers don't have to prove to the Food and Drug Administration that an herbal supplement is safe or effective before it goes on the market. You also need to be very cautious about using herbal products manufactured or bought outside the United States.

The American Diabetes Association cautions against the use of herbal supplements because little research exists to prove the remedies are safe and effective.

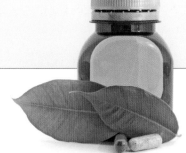

Oral drugs for type 2 diabetes

Each class of drugs that manage blood glucose works differently, and some drugs aren't for use in young children. Here are the main advantages and disadvantages — see pages 156 to 161 for more details. Your doctor may recommend one or more medications. Talk with your doctor or pharmacist before taking any over-the-counter or prescription drug. It's best to have all of your prescriptions filled at the same pharmacy so that your pharmacist can alert you to any potential drug interactions.

Drug class - Drug name (brand name)	How they work
Sulfonylureas Glimepiride (Amaryl) Glipizide (Glucotrol, Glucotrol XL) Glyburide (DiaBeta, Glynase)	Stimulate your pancreas to release more insulin
Biguanides Metformin (Fortamet, Glucophage, Glucophage XR, Riomet)	Reduce the amount of glucose your liver releases into your bloodstream between meals
Alpha-glucosidase inhibitors Acarbose (Precose) Miglitol (Glyset)	Slow absorption of glucose into your bloodstream after eating carbohydrates
Thiazolidinediones (TZDs) Pioglitazone (Actos)	Help reduce blood glucose by making body tissues more sensitive to insulin (may take a few weeks to notice effect on blood glucose)
Meglitinides Nateglinide (Starlix) Repaglinide (Prandin)	Stimulate your pancreas to release more insulin when glucose levels rise after a meal
Dipeptidyl-peptidase 4 (DPP-4) inhibitors Alogliptin (Nesina) Linagliptin (Tradjenta) Sitagliptin (Januvia) Saxagliptin (Onglyza)	Stimulate your pancreas to release more insulin when blood sugar levels rise and reduce the amount of blood sugar your liver releases into your bloodstream

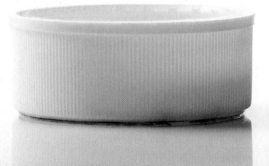

Main advantages	Main disadvantages
Work well with other oral diabetes drugs for added effectiveness to lower blood glucose	Can cause abnormally low blood glucose (hypoglycemia)
Do not cause hypoglycemia; may promote weight loss; may reduce blood fats (cholesterol and triglycerides)	Can cause nausea, upset stomach and diarrhea (typically resolves over time); rare, serious side effect is lactic acidosis (lactic acid builds up in your body)
Limit rapid rise of blood glucose that can occur after meals (taken with meals); may promote weight loss	Can cause abdominal bloating and discomfort, gas, and diarrhea, so start in smaller doses; high doses can harm your liver; less effective on lowering blood glucose than are other oral drugs
Convenient: taken once or twice a day with or without food; not linked with stomach upset when used alone	Can cause side effects such as weight gain, swelling (edema) and fluid retention that may lead to or worsen heart failure; may increase risks of bone fractures and bladder cancer; may cause liver problems; may lessen effects of birth control pills
Work quickly when taken with meals to reduce high glucose levels; less likely than sulfonylureas to cause hypoglycemia	Effects wear off quickly and drugs must be taken with each meal; can cause upset stomach and hypoglycemia
Don't cause weight gain or hypoglycemia; once-daily dosing	May cause upper respiratory tract infection, sore throat, stuffy or runny nose, or headache; may increase risk of acute pancreatitis

Alpha-glucosidase inhibitors

Alpha-glucosidase (AL-fuh-gloo-KOE-sih-days) inhibitors block the action of enzymes in the digestive tract that break down carbohydrates into glucose, delaying the digestion of carbohydrates. Glucose is absorbed into your bloodstream slower than usual, limiting the rapid rise in blood glucose that usually occurs right after a meal.

Two medications are in this class: acarbose (Precose) and miglitol (Glyset). You take them with each meal. Because these drugs aren't as effective as sulfonylureas or metformin in controlling blood glucose levels, they're typically prescribed along with other drugs to control high glucose levels after meals (postprandial elevations).

Possible side effects

Alpha-glucosidase inhibitors can cause gastrointestinal side effects, including abdominal bloating and pain, gas, and diarrhea. These effects usually occur during the first few weeks and decrease with time. If you start with a low dose and gradually increase the amount, you're more likely to have mild instead of severe symptoms.

Used alone, these drugs don't cause hypoglycemia. But when taken with another oral diabetes medication, such as a sulfonylurea, or with insulin, you run a higher risk of low blood glucose. If you do experience hypoglycemia, drink milk or use glucose tablets or gel to treat it. Don't use table sugar (sucrose) or fruit juice because alpha-glucosidase inhibitors block the absorption.

Precautions

Because of possible digestive side effects, you shouldn't take acarbose or miglitol if you have these medical conditions:

⏵ Irritable bowel syndrome
⏵ Ulcerative colitis or Crohn's disease
⏵ Partial intestinal obstruction or a predisposition for this problem
⏵ A chronic malabsorption disorder, like celiac disease
⏵ Serious kidney or liver problems

If taken in high doses, acarbose can injure your liver. Fortunately, the damage is usually reversible by reducing the dose of the medication or discontinuing it.

Thiazolidinediones (TZDs)

Many people with type 2 diabetes have a resistance to insulin that prevents insulin from working properly. Thiazolidinediones (thie-uh-zole-uh-deen-DYE-owns), also called TZDs, help reduce blood glucose by making body tissues more sensitive to insulin. As a result, less glucose remains in your bloodstream.

This class of medications includes the drugs pioglitazone (Actos) and rosiglitazone (Avandia). However, in 2010, Avandia was withdrawn from the market in Europe. Until recently, its availability was tightly restricted in the United States.

Possible side effects

Side effects from the medications may include weight gain, swelling (edema) and fluid retention. In some people, increased fluid retention leads to or worsens heart failure. Some studies also associated rosiglitazone with an increased heart attack risk.

The following signs or symptoms can indicate heart failure. Contact your doctor right away if you experience:

⏵ Shortness of breath
⏵ Trouble sleeping, such as waking up short of breath
⏵ Weakness or tiredness
⏵ Rapid weight gain (from fluid retention)
⏵ Swelling (edema) in your legs, ankles, feet

Use of TZDs use also is associated with osteoporosis with an increased risk of fractures, anemia and weight gain. Pioglitazone use also has been linked with increased risk of bladder cancer

Precautions

Taken alone, TZDs don't cause low blood glucose, but when used with a sulfonylurea or insulin, hypoglycemia can occur.

TZDs may make birth control pills less effective. In addition, for a woman who's not ovulating but hasn't yet gone through menopause, it's possible that taking a TZD could cause a start in ovulation, with risk of pregnancy.

Meglitinides

Meglitinides (meh-GLIH-tih-nides) are chemically different from sulfonylureas, but their effects are similar. These medications cause a rapid, but short-lived, release of insulin by your pancreas. Because they work quickly and their effects wear off rapidly, the medications are taken with meals. This way they kick into action shortly after eating, when your blood glucose level is highest.

Nateglinide (Starlix) and repaglinide (Prandin) are the only drugs in this class to receive Food and Drug Administration (FDA) approval. If you have liver or kidney disease, your doctor will likely take that into account when deciding if meglitinides are appropriate for you.

Possible side effects

Like sulfonylureas, meglitinides can cause low blood glucose (hypoglycemia). However, the risk of hypoglycemia with meglitinides is lower because of their short duration of action. The drugs may cause stomach upset in some people.

Precautions

If you miss a meal, skip that dose. Similar to sulfonylureas, be aware of possible drug interactions if you're taking other medications or using alcohol.

DPP-4 inhibitors

The medications, known as dipeptidyl-peptidase 4 (DPP-4) inhibitors, may be used along with diet and exercise to improve glycemic control in people with type 2 diabetes. They may also be taken as an add-on treatment in combination with another diabetes medication.

This group of medications includes alogliptin (Nesina), linagliptin (Tradjenta), saxagliptin (Onglyza) and sitagliptin (Januvia). They work by preventing the breakdown of glucagon-like peptide 1. This hormone, which is secreted by the gut, prompts insulin production after a meal — but only if blood glucose levels are high.

Possible side effects

The most common side effects of DPP-4 inhibitors are respiratory tract infection, sore throat and diarrhea. DPP-4 inhibitors are also associated with increased risk of acute pancreatitis.

Precautions

Talk to your doctor before taking this type of medication if you have kidney problems or if you're pregnant, planning to become pregnant or are breast-feeding.

What should I do if I forget to take my medication?

That depends on which drugs you take. For example, alpha-glucosidase inhibitors should only be taken with meals. If you miss a dose, you may take it if you've just finished eating — otherwise, wait until the next meal. With certain drugs, such as metformin, if you're six or more hours late, don't take it, and don't double the next dose — just continue to follow your regular medication schedule.

For specific recommendations, check the instructions that came with your prescription, or call your pharmacist or doctor for advice.

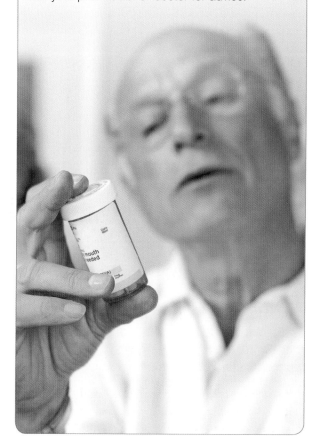

Oral drug combinations

The goal of combination therapy is to maximize the glucose-lowering effects of diabetes medications. By combining medications from different drug classes, the medications may work in two different ways to control your blood glucose. The most common combination therapy is to take two separate drugs at the same time. Two drugs also may be combined into one pill. (See Combination pills, this page.)

Some doctors prescribe three drugs at a time. More studies are necessary to determine the benefits of triple-drug therapy, but this may be an option if two oral medications don't achieve your goal.

A sulfonylurea and metformin

Sulfonylureas are often the base of combination therapy because of their ability to boost and maintain insulin secretion. A sulfonylurea combined with metformin is the most extensively studied drug combination. The medications seem to work more effectively together than they do individually. Metformin can help people who are overweight avoid additional weight gain and, in some cases, lose weight. Side effects of this drug combination include nausea, diarrhea and risk of low blood glucose.

A sulfonylurea and a TZD

Adding a TZD medication to a sulfonylurea may help when the maximum dose of a sulfonylurea isn't working for you, you're overweight, and your cells are highly insulin resistant. This combination also increases your risk of low blood glucose because TZDs improve your body's use of insulin stimulated by sulfonylureas. This combination also increases the risk of weight gain

Metformin and a DPP-4 inhibitor

A combination of metformin and a DPP-4 inhibitor is effective in controlling blood glucose without increasing risks of low blood glucose (hypoglycemia).

Possible side effects from combining metformin and an alpha-glucosidase inhibitor are the same as those for the individual drugs.

Combination pills

Most combination therapies involve taking two separate drugs. However, the FDA has approved four types of combination pills:
- Glipizide-metformin (Metaglip)
- Glyburide-metformin (Glucovance)
- Rosiglitazone-metformin (Avandamet)
- Sitagliptin-metformin (Janumet)

Although combination pills are convenient because you take fewer pills, there are trade-offs. For example, if you have a side effect, it's harder to tell which medication may be causing it. But if you took two separate pills, the doctor could advise cutting back on one at a time to see which one is linked with the side effect. In addition, these combination pills can cost more than the two pills taken separately.

Metformin and a TZD

The TZD pioglitazone is approved by the Food and Drug Administration (FDA) for use with metformin. The combination therapy is more effective at reducing blood glucose than is either medication alone. Precautions and side effects are the same as those listed for each drug.

Oral drugs and insulin

Combining insulin with an oral medication can help both drugs work more effectively. The combination can also lower your daily insulin requirements and may limit weight gain associated with insulin therapy alone.

A sulfonylurea and insulin

Adding a dose of insulin at bedtime to your regular dosage of a sulfonylurea may improve blood glucose control. At first glance, a sulfonylurea and insulin don't appear to be a likely combination because they both boost insulin levels. However, they promote the circulation of insulin in different parts of your body. Using a sulfonylurea with insulin may allow you to use lower doses of insulin and achieve the same control.

This therapy — called bedtime insulin, daytime sulfonylurea (BIDS) — may be useful if a combination of a sulfonylurea and metformin hasn't worked for you.

Metformin and insulin

Similar to a sulfonylurea combination, combining metformin with insulin can help reduce your insulin dose. Metformin helps your liver become more sensitive to insulin, making better use of it. Metformin also counteracts the problem of weight gain associated with insulin use. In fact, you may actually lose weight when using this combination.

An alpha-glucosidase inhibitor and insulin

Acarbose, an alpha-glucosidase inhibitor, is approved by the FDA for use with insulin. Acarbose slows the absorption of carbohydrates, which may reduce your daily need for insulin, but this also increases risk of low blood glucose that can occur with insulin therapy.

A TZD and insulin

If your blood glucose is well-controlled, a TZD with insulin can reduce your daily insulin needs. If you have trouble controlling your blood glucose, adding a TZD may help better regulate your blood glucose. However, this combination isn't recommended because it can cause significant weight gain.

Side effects include low blood glucose and increased risk of fluid retention and heart failure in some people, along with the side effects of TZDs.

Insulin and type 2 diabetes

Insulin is always needed for treating type 1 diabetes, but it's also an effective medication for treating type 2 diabetes. You may take insulin alone, or you may use it in combination with an oral diabetes medication. Your doctor may recommend insulin injections if you have poor control of your diabetes, because either your pancreas isn't making enough insulin or you aren't responding to other medications. Your doctor also may turn first to insulin if:

▶ Your fasting blood glucose level is markedly high — more than 300 milligrams per deciliter (mg/dL) — and you have a high level of ketones in your urine

▶ You have a markedly high fasting blood glucose level and are experiencing signs and symptoms of diabetes, such as excessive thirst and frequent urination

▶ You have gestational diabetes that can't be controlled by diet

You may need to take insulin for a short period to help bring your diabetes under control during an illness, or you may use the medication long term to keep your blood glucose in a safe range.

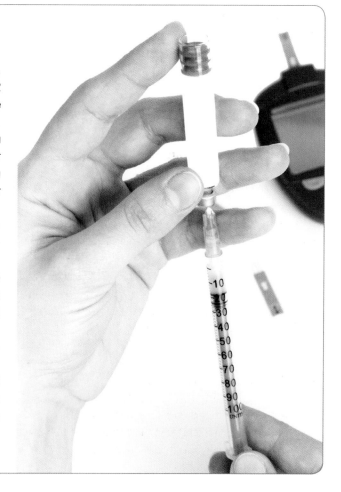

Injectable drugs

Although not used as commonly as oral medications, injectable drugs provide additional options for treating type 2 diabetes.

Exenatide

Exenatide (Byetta, Bydureon) belongs to a class of drugs called incretin mimetics, which mimic the action of human hormones called incretins. Byetta comes in a pre-filled pen and is injected twice daily under the skin of your thigh, abdomen or upper arm. Bydureon, a long-acting version of the drug, only needs to be injected once a week.

Exenatide mimics the action of a hormone secreted by the gut — glucagon-like peptide 1 (GLP-1) — which prompts insulin production after a meal, but only if blood glucose levels are high. This differs from current drugs, which promote insulin production regardless of blood glucose level.

Exenatide also reduces appetite and the release of the hormone glucagon, which would otherwise raise blood glucose after meals. Exenatide also may slow stomach emptying.

Exenatide is used with metformin or a sulfonylurea, or a combination of the two. Exenatide may decrease your appetite, so you may eat less, resulting in modest weight loss.

Possible side effects

The most common side effect of exenatide is nausea, which often improves with time. Other side effects include vomiting, diarrhea, dizziness, headache and an acidic stomach. Exenatide taken with a sulfonylurea increases the risk of hypoglycemia. Lowering the dose of sulfonylurea may reduce this risk. Exenatide is also associated with increased risk of acute pancreatitis and altered kidney function.

Liraglutide

Like exenatide, liraglutide (Victoza) stimulates insulin production by mimicking some actions of the hormone GLP-1. The drug stimulates insulin production when blood glucose levels rise, reduces the release of glucagon and may slow stomach emptying. Liraglutide may also decrease appetite.

Liraglutide comes in a pre-filled pen and is injected once a day. Like exenatide, liraglutide is used in combination with first line"medications, such as metformin.

Possible side effects

The most common side effects are nausea, diarrhea and vomiting. The drug has been linked with an increased risk of acute pancreatitis.

Pramlintide

The first in a new class of drugs called amylin mimetics, pramlintide (Symlin) mimics the action of the human hormone amylin, produced by the pancreas.

Using a needle and syringe, you can inject pramlintide into your stomach area (abdomen) or your thigh immediately before meals, along with rapid-acting insulin (in a separate syringe). This slows down the movement of food through your stomach after meals. As a result, it affects how rapidly glucose enters your bloodstream.

Pramlintide also appears to be linked with modest weight loss. Pramlintide is designed for adults with type 1 or type 2 diabetes who require insulin and aren't reaching their target blood glucose levels.

Possible side effects

The most common side effect of pramlintide is nausea, which usually improves over time. Other side effects include vomiting, abdominal pain, headache, fatigue and dizziness.

In addition, pramlintide is linked with an increased risk of severe insulin-induced hypoglycemia (seen within three hours of injection), particularly in people with type 1 diabetes. Severe hypoglycemia makes it difficult to think clearly or drive.

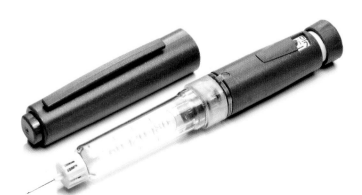

Kidney dialysis

Good control of your blood sugar (glucose) levels and blood pressure are two key factors in helping to prevent kidney problems. Over several years, long-term kidney disease can lead to chronic kidney failure (end-stage renal disease), which is a serious, life-threatening condition. This is when your kidneys can no longer remove harmful wastes from your blood and your body retains extra fluid.

Whether you have type 1 or type 2 diabetes, when your kidneys fail to work properly, you have two treatment options: Kidney dialysis or a kidney transplant. Many people need dialysis while they're waiting for a kidney transplant.

There are other types of transplantation, including pancreas and islet cell transplants, that attempt to restore insulin production in people with diabetes.

The evaluation for any type of transplant — kidney or otherwise — will assess whether you:

▶ Are healthy enough to have surgery and tolerate lifelong post-transplant medications
▶ Have a medical condition that would make a transplant unlikely to succeed
▶ Are willing and able to take medications as directed
▶ Are strong enough emotionally to tolerate the typical long wait for a donor organ and have family and friends who are supportive to help during this stressful time

What is kidney dialysis?

Kidney dialysis is an artificial means of removing waste products and extra fluid from your blood when your kidneys can no longer do this. There are two main types of dialysis: hemodialysis and peritoneal dialysis.

Hemodialysis

The most common form of dialysis is hemodialysis. It filters your blood through an artificial kidney (dialyzer) to remove extra fluids, chemicals and wastes. Blood is pumped out of your body to the artificial kidney through an access point (surgically created from your own blood vessels or a piece of tubing), usually in your arm.

Surgery to create the access point is usually done a couple of months before you're set to start dialysis, to allow time for healing. Most people need treatment three times a week, with about three to five hours for each session. This is usually done in a dialysis center, but it can be done at home if you have someone to help you.

During dialysis, you may have side effects, such as unstable or low blood pressure, cramps, or an upset stomach. Together with hemodialysis, medications (such as blood thinners, blood pressure medications and iron supplements) and a special diet will round out your treatment plan.

Peritoneal dialysis

This type of dialysis uses the network of tiny blood vessels in your abdomen (peritoneal cavity) to filter your blood. First, a surgeon implants a small, flexible tube (catheter) into your abdomen and allows healing time. Then you're ready to use one of the methods described below.

With both methods, a dialysis solution is infused into and drained out of your abdomen to remove waste, chemicals and extra water. Each cycle is called an exchange. You can be more independent with peritoneal dialysis because you don't have to travel to a dialysis center. The main potential complications of peritoneal dialysis are infections, weight gain and hernia.

Continuous ambulatory peritoneal dialysis (CAPD)

Ambulatory refers to on the go. CAPD can be done at home, work or any clean place — you perform the exchanges by hand instead of using a machine. Each exchange takes about 30 to 40 minutes, and it's done four or five times each day. You can do your normal activities between exchanges.

Continuous cycling peritoneal dialysis (CCPD)

Also called automated peritoneal dialysis, CCPD involves a machine that automatically infuses the cleansing fluid into your peritoneal cavity and drains it several times during the night while you sleep. This allows your days to be free, but you need to be attached to the machine at night for 10 to 12 hours.

Both CAPD and CCPD

If you weigh more than 175 pounds or waste is filtered slowly within your body, you may need a combination of CAPD and CCPD to get the right dialysis dose.

Drawbacks

Dialysis can dramatically change your lifestyle because of the frequent treatments needed. You'll also have to follow a special diet to manage your intake of protein, liquids, salt (sodium), potassium and phosphorus.

With peritoneal dialysis, you must be careful about your technique to prevent serious abdominal infection at the opening where the catheter enters your abdomen. In addition, many people on dialysis are prone to sleep disorders, bone problems, fluid build-up and other serious conditions.

A kidney transplant offers the best chance to restore normal kidney function and a more regular lifestyle. It also offers improved odds for long-term survival, but it's not without risks and there are long waiting lists.

During hemodialysis (right), a needle is inserted into your arm through a special access point. Your blood is then directed through the needle and special tubing to a machine called a dialyzer, which filters your blood a few ounces at a time. The filtered blood returns to your body through another needle. While undergoing treatment you can read, watch television, take a nap or do other sedentary activities. Some people use this time to catch up on phone calls.

Access point care

Before you start hemodialysis, a surgeon creates an access point for blood to leave your body for cleansing and then re-enter your body during treatment. To prevent injury and infection at the access point:

- Keep the area clean
- Don't use the arm with the access point for blood pressure readings or to draw blood samples not associated with the dialysis treatment
- Don't lift heavy objects or put pressure on the arm with the access point
- Don't cover the access point with tight clothing or jewelry
- Check the pulse in the access point every day
- Don't sleep with the access arm under your head or body

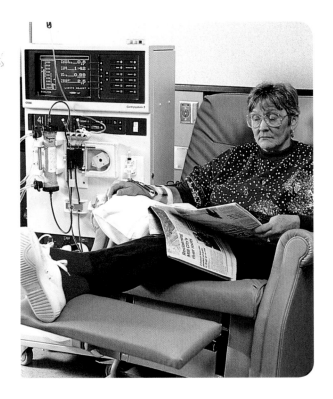

Kidney transplant

A successful transplant won't cure kidney disease due to diabetes, but it can restore sufficient kidney function and help you feel better so that you have a better quality of life. It also frees you from dialysis.

Types of kidney transplants

There are two types of kidney transplants. You may receive a kidney from a deceased donor or have a living-donor transplant.

Because few people sign up to be living donors, it's more common to get a kidney from a deceased donor. The donor-recipient matching system considers blood type, tissue type and an antibody test (crossmatch), which determines whether the recipient has antibodies to the potential donor. A transplant from a living donor has some advantages:

▶ If a donor is related by birth, you have a better chance of a good match.
▶ It's easier to evaluate the health of the donor and donor organ.
▶ You don't have to place your name on a national waiting list.
▶ Surgery can be scheduled in advance at an optimal time for donor and recipient, rather than being scheduled without advance notice upon the death of a donor.

Surgery and follow-up

The damaged kidney will most likely not be removed, and the surgeon will place the new kidney in your lower abdomen. The blood vessels of the new kidney will be attached to blood vessels in the lower part of your abdomen, just above one of your legs. The tube that links the new kidney to the bladder (ureter) will be connected to your bladder.

Even with the best possible match between you and the donor, your immune system will try to reject the new kidney. Your drug regimen will include immunosuppressive drugs — drugs that suppress the activity of your immune system. You'll likely take these medications for the rest of your life.

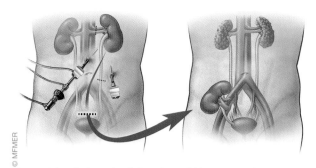

In a minimally invasive living-donor kidney transplant, surgeons use small incisions to remove the kidney from its donor and insert it in the recipient.

The drugs may cause side effects, such as a round and full face, weight gain, acne, facial hair, and stomach problems. These effects may decrease as time goes on. Some immunosuppressive drugs can raise the risk of developing or worsening conditions such as high blood pressure, high cholesterol and cancer.

Because immunosuppressive drugs make your body more vulnerable to infection, your doctor may also prescribe antibacterial, antiviral and anti-fungal medications. Treatment becomes a balancing act between preventing rejection and managing side effects.

Other transplant procedures

Researchers hope to one day find a treatment to prevent or halt diabetes. They're still a long way from a cure.

Two types of surgery, however, can help some individuals eliminate the need for daily insulin injections: pancreas transplant and islet cell transplant.

Pancreas transplant

A pancreas transplant is a treatment option if you have diabetes and are in kidney failure (also requiring a kidney transplant) or you don't respond well to standard insulin treatments.

A successful pancreas transplant means either insulin is no longer needed for control of blood glucose or you stop having serious low and high blood glucose episodes. However, it's far from a cure. There are life-threatening risks, especially if you have heart and blood vessel disease.

A transplant center will evaluate you to see if you meet the eligibility requirements, including medical and emotional factors, similar to the criteria for a kidney transplant.

Several different types of transplants involve the pancreas. Blood type, tissue type and an antibody test are key factors in the success of all types of pancreas transplants. Most pancreas transplants involve transplanting a whole pancreas from a deceased donor.

Kidney-pancreas transplants

More than half of all pancreas transplants are performed at the same time as a kidney transplant. The strategy is to give you a healthy kidney and pancreas to reduce the potential for future diabetes-related kidney damage. In most cases, the organs come from the same deceased donor. This dual transplant appears to contribute to better survival for both organs.

Pancreas-after-kidney transplants

You may receive a pancreas transplant after you've had a successful kidney transplant. The treatment goal is similar to a kidney-pancreas transplant. The normal insulin function of your new pancreas should decrease the potential for diabetes-related kidney damage.

Pancreas-only transplants

Pancreas-only transplants (also called pancreas-alone transplants) are performed when there's normal or near-normal kidney function. Your doctor may recommend this option if you have frequent insulin reactions or poor blood glucose control despite the best efforts to manage your disease.

If your insulin treatment and other disease management strategies are working, a pancreas-only transplant is most likely not a good option. A study reported in 2003 indicated that people with working kidneys who received pancreas-only transplants had significantly lower survival rates than did those who used insulin and other conventional treatments. A

pancreas that's transplanted along with a kidney is less likely to fail than a pancreas-only transplant.

Pancreas islet cell transplants

An experimental procedure called a pancreas islet cell transplant can provide new insulin-producing cells from a donor pancreas rather than a whole organ. As this procedure is improved, it could become a viable option for people with type 1 diabetes (see below).

Surgery and follow-up

During surgery, your own pancreas will most likely not be removed. The surgeon will transplant the new pancreas with a small portion of the donor's small intestine still attached into your lower abdominal cavity. Your new pancreas should start working immediately, and your old pancreas will continue to perform its other functions.

Post-transplant treatment is a balancing act between preventing rejection and managing side effects. The results of pancreas transplants vary by the expertise and experience of the transplant center, as well as factors such as the age and health of the candidate and the condition of the donated organ.

Islet cell transplant

As mentioned earlier, another procedure called pancreas islet cell transplant shows much promise as a treatment option for some people with type 1 diabetes. With this transplant procedure, only the hormone-producing cells (islets) from a donor pancreas, rather than the entire organ, are transplanted into your body.

Throughout the pancreas are clusters of specialized cells (islets of Langerhans), which produce insulin. In type 1 diabetes, the body's immune system, which normally protects the body from viruses and bacteria, attacks and kills the islet cells.

An islet cell transplant has some of the same benefits as a pancreas transplant, but is a less invasive surgery. However, the transplanted islets do not survive as long as the whole pancreas transplant. There also are risks associated with the procedure. As more people participate in clinical trials of this type of transplant, a clearer picture of its safety, long-term effects and potential as a treatment option will emerge.

How does it work?

Current procedures for islet cell transplants are based largely on standards (protocols) developed by the National Institutes of Health (NIH). The NIH group that developed the procedures included researchers from multiple islet cell transplant centers.

After a donor organ has been transferred to a transplant center, lab technicians extract only the islet cells and purify them. A specialist called an interventional radiologist or a surgeon performs the islet cell transplant through a minimally invasive procedure.

Using image-guided methods, the radiologist or transplant surgeon directs a tube through an opening in your abdomen to the blood vessel leading into your liver (portal vein). The islet cells are infused through this tube to your liver. The cells spread throughout the liver, attaching to small blood vessels. The liver is a good site for the transplant because it's easier to get to than your pancreas is, and the islet cells seem to do well in that location.

About a million islets are needed for a transplant to be effective in an average-sized person. As donor organs become available, more cell infusions are done until the desired insulin production is reached.

Your body will regard the new cells as it would a new organ. So a successful transplant depends on a treatment regimen that includes immunosuppressive drugs. In addition, the availability of islet cells is very limited because of the shortage of organ donors.

How effective is it?

In 2001, the National Institute of Diabetes and Digestive and Kidney Diseases established the Collaborative Islet Transplant Registry (CITR) to collect and analyze data on islet cell transplants performed at centers in the United States and Canada.

The CITR's 2010 annual report presented data on 571 individuals. During the first year after their final infusions, about 60 percent no longer needed to take insulin. By the end of the second year, the percentage of participants who remained insulin independent dropped to approximately 50 percent. However, long-term insulin independence is difficult to maintain, and eventually most recipients needed to start taking insulin again.

The NIH has sponsored a clinical trial to study islet cell transplantation. Results are expected by 2014. After that, islet cell transplantation may become more widely available for people with type 1 diabetes.

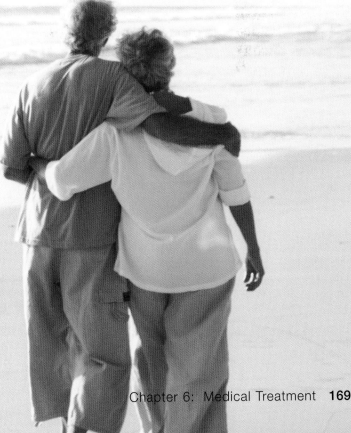

Chapter 7
Staying Healthy

Yearly checkups 173

Important tests you should have 174

Caring for your eyes 179

Caring for your feet 180

Caring for your teeth 183

Getting vaccinated 184

Managing stress 184

Preparing for pregnancy 190

Understanding menstruation and diabetes 195

Dealing with menopause 195

Living with erectile dysfunction 196

A visit with Dr. Steven Smith

"Staying healthy and reducing your risks of chronic disease is like riding a bicycle. ...You are the one that provides the energy to better health by pedaling the self-management wheel."

Staying healthy and reducing your risks of chronic disease is like riding a bicycle. It involves implementing effective self-management behaviors to prevent or slow the progression of complications. The self-management wheel for diabetes includes nutrition, exercise, medications, self-monitoring, problem-solving, risk reduction and psychosocial adjustment.

It may seem at times that you're riding a unicycle, but in fact it is a bicycle. You are the one that provides the energy to better health by pedaling the self-management wheel. The bicycle's frame is important in supporting your self-management efforts. It includes family, friends, work and the health care system influencing your day-to-day decisions. Your health care provider and team are the front wheel. They provide guidance and direction, but they don't provide the energy. It's up to you to pedal the bike.

Members of your health care team are experts in helping you set realistic goals, and they act as the guiding front wheel. The framework of the bike that connects you to your health care team often leads to collaboration and productive interactions.

This chapter emphasizes the importance of regular checkups and preventive care. Creating an action

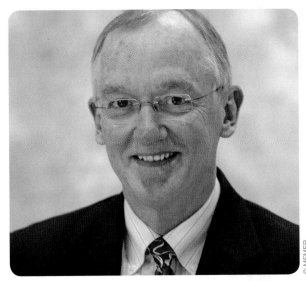

Steven A. Smith, M.D.
Endocrinology

plan is a good way to start. Make certain the plan is realistic and can be part of your life. Periodically, reassess that action plan and ask yourself, "Am I still meeting the goals that I set?" If not, problem solve with family, friends and your health care team to help redirect your pedaling efforts.

"Life is like riding a bicycle: You don't fall off unless you stop pedaling."— Claude Pepper

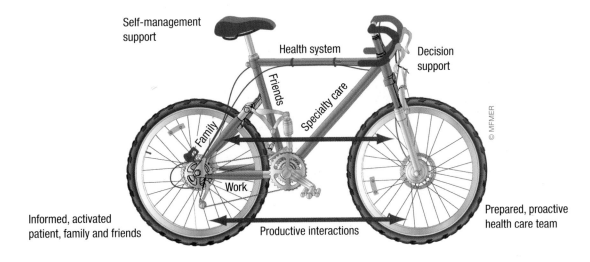

Your health care team

Successful management of diabetes usually involves working with several professionals. Your health care team may include the following:

▶ **Primary doctor.** Look for a doctor who specializes in diabetes, such as a board-certified endocrinologist.

▶ **Nurse.** A nurse, preferably a certified diabetes educator (explained at right), can help you learn more about your diabetes and counsel you on self-care.

▶ **Registered dietitian.** A registered dietitian can work with you to develop a healthy-eating plan to help control your blood glucose levels.

▶ **Eye doctor.** An eye doctor (ophthalmologist or optometrist) who has expertise in diabetes-related eye problems can help detect early eye disease.

▶ **Foot doctor.** A foot doctor (podiatrist) who has expertise in diabetes-related foot problems can detect and treat foot problems, such as calluses or sores, and help you learn how to prevent future problems.

▶ **Other professionals.** Depending on your needs, you may also benefit from seeing a kidney specialist (nephrologist), nerve specialist (neurologist) or a mental health professional. Look for individuals who have experience in working with people who have diabetes.

What is a certified diabetes educator?

A certified diabetes educator (C.D.E.) is a professional who has passed a national exam on diabetes education and is certified to teach people with diabetes how to manage their disease. Although a C.D.E. is often a registered nurse or a registered dietitian, other professionals, such as physicians, physician assistants and pharmacists, also may be certified.

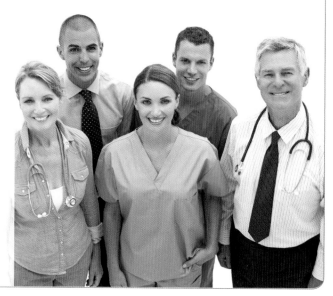

Within weeks to months after your diagnosis, managing your diabetes should start to become routine. You'll gradually develop a pattern for testing your blood sugar (glucose), taking your medications, exercising and eating.

But you often may wonder, "How am I doing?" You'd like to know if your efforts at controlling your blood glucose are paying off.

You can find out the answer by keeping in regular contact with your health care team and making sure you receive appropriate tests during your checkups. These tests can assess how well you're doing in controlling your blood glucose and spot potential problems or complications that may arise. Regular checkups also provide an opportunity to hear suggestions from your health care team on how to meet your goals.

How often you should see your doctor or other members of your health care team depends on what's happening with your health. If you're having trouble keeping your blood glucose levels down or if you're changing medication, you may need to contact a member of your health care team weekly. You may even need to check in more often.

In general, though, if you're feeling good and keeping your blood glucose within the range that you and your doctor have agreed upon, you probably won't need to see your doctor more than four times a year. If you reach and are able to maintain your blood glucose goals, the visits may be less often.

Yearly checkups

Even if your diabetes is under control, it's important you see your doctor at least once a year. During a yearly checkup, your doctor can check for potential complications and the two of you can discuss how your treatment plan is working.

What to expect

Your doctor will likely begin your exam by asking you questions about your blood glucose readings and overall health:

▶ How have you been feeling?
▶ Have you been experiencing any new symptoms or problems?
▶ Have you been able to keep your blood glucose within your target range?

It's important to bring your daily log of blood glucose readings with you to your appointment so that your doctor can review it. Many doctors' offices are also using technology to access glucose meter results to help in the discussion. Any episodes of high or low blood glucose should be discussed to try to determine what may have caused them.

Other issues you may want to cover with your doctor or a diabetes educator include:

▶ Temporary adjustments you made to your treatment program, including changes in medication, to accommodate for high or low blood glucose readings
▶ Problems you may be having in following your treatment program
▶ Emotional and social problems you may be experiencing
▶ Changes in your use of tobacco or alcohol

During your checkup, a member of your health care team may also do checks of your blood pressure, weight, feet and urine.

Check your blood pressure

High blood pressure (hypertension) can damage your blood vessels, and you're already at increased risk of blood vessel disease if you have diabetes. Diabetes and high blood pressure are often associated, and when present together they significantly increase your risk of complications. Controlling high blood pressure can help prevent complications.

Check your weight

If you have diabetes and you're overweight or obese, losing weight can help you control your blood glucose — gaining more weight will make it harder to manage your glucose. If you take a diabetes medication, weight loss may reduce your need for medication.

Check your feet

At each visit you should have a brief examination of your feet. At least once a year you should have a thorough foot exam. During a thorough exam, here's what your doctor is looking for:

▶ Breaks in the skin, which could lead to an infection
▶ Pulses in your foot, which indicate if you have good blood circulation in the foot, and a sense of touch, which indicates if sensory nerves in the foot are working properly

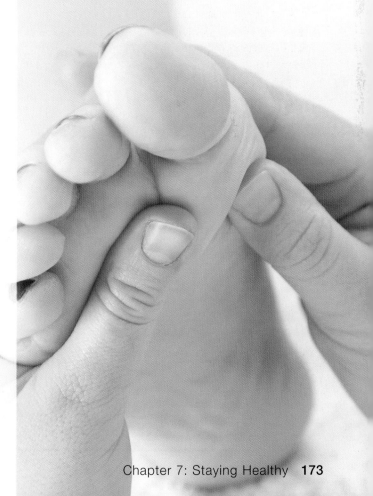

- Normal range of motion, to make sure there is no muscle or bone damage
- Bony deformations or evidence of increased pressure, such as calluses, which may indicate that you need different shoes

If a problem is identified, examine your feet regularly to make sure the condition doesn't worsen. If you're unable to examine your feet yourself, recruit the help of a family member or a close friend.

Request blood and urine tests

Simple blood and urine tests can detect early signs of diabetes complications, such as kidney disease. The earlier you discover and treat emerging problems, the better your chances of stopping, or at least slowing, the damage.

Important tests you should have

The following four tests are especially important to people with diabetes. Three of them examine your blood, and one checks your urine.

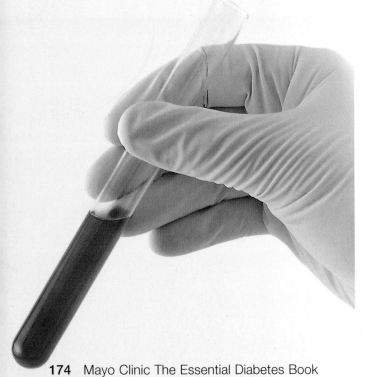

A1C test

An A1C test, also known as a glycated hemoglobin test, is an effective tool for determining how well you're managing your blood sugar (glucose). This blood test is different from a fasting blood glucose test or a daily finger stick, both of which only measure your blood glucose at any given moment. An A1C test indicates your average blood glucose level over the past two to three months.

How it works

Some of the glucose in your bloodstream attaches to hemoglobin, a protein found in red blood cells. This is known as glycated hemoglobin (A1C).

To check your A1C level, blood is usually drawn from a vein in your arm, and the sample is sent to a lab for analysis. Although some home test kits are available, it's important that this test be done correctly. Test results indicate what percentage of your hemoglobin is sugarcoated (glycated).

Normal ranges may vary between laboratories, but most commonly:

- For people who do not have diabetes, 4 to 5.6 percent is normal.
- A level of 5.7 to 6.4 percent indicates prediabetes. Or if you have been previously diagnosed with diabetes, it indicates good control of your blood sugar.
- Less than 7 percent is an ideal goal for most people with diabetes.
- More than 8 percent is a concern and may indicate a need for a change in your treatment plan

Talk with your doctor to find out your specific goal. Although an A1C level under 7 percent is a common target, your doctor may recommend a level as close to 6 percent as possible if you're pregnant or you need a stricter goal for other reasons. Less than 8 percent is appropriate for people at risk of low blood sugar levels.

If you've had testing done elsewhere and you're seeing a new doctor, it's important that your doctor take this possible variation into account when interpreting your test results.

How often should you have it done?

If your therapy has recently changed or you're not meeting your blood glucose goals, your doctor will likely recommend an A1C test every three months. If you're able to control your blood glucose levels and meet treatment goals, an A1C test is recommended at least twice a year.

How does it help?

An A1C test can help in many ways. Say, for instance, you're having trouble maintaining a normal blood glucose level and your doctor is deciding whether to prescribe medication or allow more time for you to improve your diet and exercise plan. Your doctor may have you increase the amount of time you exercise for two or three months and then have you come in for another A1C test. If the test shows an improved reading, then increased exercise may be all that you need to control your blood glucose, and your doctor may not prescribe medication.

In addition, the test is a way to alert you and your doctor to potential problems. If you've had normal A1C readings for several months or years and suddenly you have an abnormal reading, this may be a sign that your treatment plan needs a change, including more frequent blood glucose testing. Results of the A1C test also indicate your risk of complications from diabetes — the higher your test result is, the greater your risk.

Lipid panel

A lipid panel measures the fats (lipids) in your blood, including cholesterol and triglycerides. Blood is drawn from a vein in your arm and sent to a lab. To get an accurate reading, it's best to fast for nine to 12 hours before blood is drawn.

The measurements can indicate your risk of having a heart attack or other heart disease. The panel typically includes:

◗ **Low-density lipoprotein (LDL) cholesterol.** This "bad" cholesterol promotes accumulation of fatty deposits (plaques) in your arteries. These plaques reduce blood supply to the heart and other vital organs.
◗ **High-density lipoprotein (HDL) cholesterol.** This "good" cholesterol helps protect against heart disease by helping clear excess cholesterol from your body. This keeps your arteries open and your blood circulating more freely.

◗ **Triglycerides.** A normal amount of these blood fats is needed for good health to help your body store fat that's later used for energy. But high levels of triglycerides increase your risk of heart and blood vessel disease.
◗ **Total cholesterol.** This is the sum of your blood's LDL cholesterol, HDL cholesterol and a portion of triglycerides. Higher levels may put you at greater risk of heart and blood vessel disease.

How often should you have it done?

People who don't have diabetes need a lipid panel at least every five years — more often if their blood-fat levels are above normal or they have a family history of elevated blood fats.

If you have diabetes, you should have a lipid panel at least once a year, but more often if you're not achieving your lipid goals.

If your lipid values are at low-risk levels — LDL less than 100 milligrams per deciliter (mg/dL), HDL higher than 50 mg/dL, triglycerides under 150 mg/dL — a lipid panel every two years may be enough.

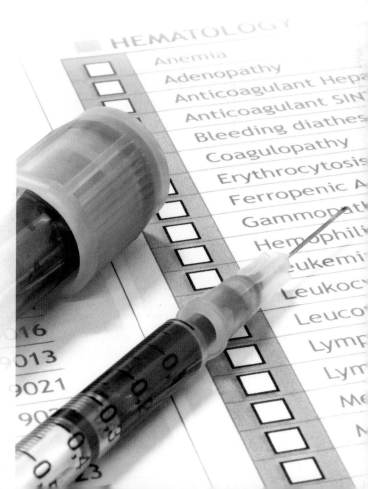

However, if you have cardiovascular disease, your doctor may recommend a goal of less than 70 mg/dL for LDL cholesterol with the use of a cholesterol-lowering drug called a statin. Talk with your doctor about your target lipid goal.

How does it help?

A rising level of blood fats can alert your doctor to increased risk of blood vessel damage. That's because diabetes can accelerate the development of clogged and hardened arteries (atherosclerosis), which increases your risk of a heart attack, stroke, and poor circulation in your feet and legs.

Knowing your blood-fat levels also helps your doctor determine if you might benefit from medication to help lower your cholesterol or triglyceride levels.

Diet and exercise are the first defenses against unhealthy blood-fat levels, just as they are in managing diabetes. Your doctor may prescribe lipid-lowering medication if these steps aren't effective or if your LDL or triglyceride levels are above your target goals.

Serum creatinine test

A serum creatinine (kree-AT-ih-nin) test measures the level of creatinine in your blood and can alert you and your doctors to kidney problems.

Creatinine is a waste byproduct of creatine, a protein that supplies energy for muscle contraction. Your blood normally produces a small but relatively constant amount of creatinine. If the creatinine level in your blood rises above normal, it's a sign that your kidneys have been damaged and aren't able to function properly (renal insufficiency). The higher the creatinine level, the more advanced the kidney disease.

Normal values of serum creatinine vary, depending on your sex, muscle mass and other factors, so ask your doctor what's normal for you. Different labs may have slightly different normal ranges.

At Mayo Clinic, normal ranges are:

) 0.9 to 1.4 mg/dL for men
) 0.7 to 1.2 mg/dL for women

How often should you have it done?

You should have a serum creatinine test once a year.

Urine testing at home

Different types of home urine test kits are available, but they vary in quality — and some types aren't reliable. Depending on the kit, you can test for:
) Ketones
) Glucose and ketones
) Microscopic amounts of protein (microalbuminuria)

Ketone kits, also available in strip form, detect some ketones, but not all of them. Ketone test strips reveal results through color changes.

Some doctors recommend checks for microalbuminuria in which you mail a urine sample to a lab. A doctor must interpret the results. Ask your doctor for more information.

If you have known kidney damage or you're taking medications that could have a harmful effect on your kidneys, your doctor may recommend that you have this test more often.

How does it help?

Knowing the health of your kidneys is important because kidney function influences many decisions regarding your medical care, including which medications are safe for you to take and how aggressive to be in controlling your blood pressure.

Urine test for protein

A urine test that detects tiny amounts of protein (albumin), called a urine microalbumin test, also is used to assess kidney health.

When your kidneys are functioning normally, they filter out wastes in your blood. These wastes are removed through urination. Protein and other helpful substances remain in the bloodstream. When your kidneys become damaged, the opposite occurs — waste products remain in your blood and protein leaks into your urine.

The preferred method to screen for protein leakage is the spot collection, using about the same amount of urine provided during routine urine testing (urinalysis). This easy collection, done at a medical visit, generally provides accurate information.

An alternative method is to save all of your urine over a 24-hour period in a jug that you get from your doctor. You then return the urine jug to your doctor's office, where it's sent to a lab and analyzed.

When your kidneys first begin to leak, typically only tiny amounts of protein escape. More-advanced stages can occur after you've had diabetes for many years.

Typically, here's what your urine test results will mean, measured as milligrams (mg) of protein leakage:

▶ Less than 30 mg is normal
▶ 30 to 299 mg indicates early-stage kidney disease (microalbuminuria)
▶ 300 mg or more indicates advanced kidney disease (macroalbuminuria)

Protein in the urine can occur for reasons other than diabetes, so if your test results are higher than normal, you may be tested again to confirm that you have kidney disease.

How often should you have it done?

You should have a urine protein test once a year, starting five years after the diagnosis of type 1 diabetes or when type 2 diabetes is diagnosed. The test is also recommended during pregnancy for women with diabetes.

How does it help?

A urine test for protein can alert you and your doctor to kidney damage. By keeping your blood glucose level within a normal or near-normal range, you can help prevent the progression of kidney disease.

Controlling high blood pressure also is important in preventing further kidney damage. Blood pressure medications called angiotensin-converting enzyme (ACE) inhibitors often are prescribed to people with kidney damage because they help protect kidney function.

Other classes of blood pressure drugs also can be beneficial, and you may need more than one type.

Eating a low-protein diet may improve protein leakage by reducing the workload on your kidneys. Your diabetes educator can give you advice on a low-protein diet if you need one.

Exams, tests and quick checks

If you have diabetes, you'll need regular exams and tests to watch for current or potential health problems. Test results may indicate a need to change your treatment plan.

Which tests	How often
Blood pressure check	At every visit with your doctor
Weight check	At every visit with your doctor
Foot exam	Brief check at every visit with your doctor; thorough exam at least once a year
Eye exam	At least once a year, but more often if you have eye problems, poorly controlled diabetes, high blood pressure, kidney disease, or you're pregnant
A1C test (glycated hemoglobin test)	At least two times a year if you're meeting treatment goals and blood glucose is stable; about every three months if you're not meeting glucose goals or your treatment changed
Lipid panel (cholesterol and triglyceride levels)	At least once a year, but more often if needed to achieve your goals; every two years if lipid values are at low-risk levels (LDL less than 100 mg/dL, HDL higher than 40 mg/dL for men and higher than 50 mg/dL for women, triglycerides under 150 mg/dL)
Serum creatinine test	Once a year, but more often if you have kidney disease or are taking medications that could have a harmful effect on your kidneys
Urine test for protein (urine microalbumin test)	Once a year, starting five years after the diagnosis of type 1 diabetes, or starting when type 2 diabetes is diagnosed (also recommended during pregnancy for women with diabetes)

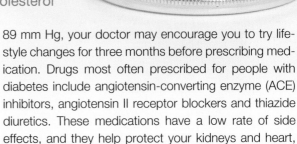

Blood relatives:
Pay attention to your blood pressure and blood cholesterol

In addition to monitoring your blood glucose, you also need to pay attention to your blood pressure and blood cholesterol.

Monitor your blood pressure

People with diabetes are about twice as likely to develop high blood pressure as are individuals who don't have diabetes. Having both diabetes and high blood pressure is serious. Similar to diabetes, high blood pressure can damage your blood vessels. When you have both of these conditions and they're not under control, you increase your risk of a heart attack, stroke or other life-threatening complications.

Blood pressure is a measure of the force of circulating blood against the walls of your arteries. The higher your blood pressure, the harder your heart has to work to pump blood to all parts of your body. Blood pressure is measured as two numbers, such as 120/70 millimeters of mercury (mm Hg). The first number (upper number) is your peak pressure at the moment your heart contracts and pumps blood (systolic pressure). The second number (lower number) is the level of pressure when your heart relaxes to allow blood to flow into your heart (diastolic pressure).

Blood pressure goals and treatment

Adults with diabetes should keep their blood pressure below 140/80 mm Hg. If you have kidney disease, your doctor may recommend a lower blood pressure. The same healthy habits that can improve your blood glucose — a balanced diet and regular exercise — can help reduce your blood pressure. If you can't control your blood pressure with diet and exercise alone, your doctor may prescribe blood pressure lowering medication.

The American Diabetes Association recommends drug therapy if your systolic pressure is at or higher than 140 mm Hg or your diastolic pressure is at or higher than 90 mm Hg. If your systolic blood pressure is 130 to 139 mm Hg or your diastolic blood pressure is 80 to 89 mm Hg, your doctor may encourage you to try lifestyle changes for three months before prescribing medication. Drugs most often prescribed for people with diabetes include angiotensin-converting enzyme (ACE) inhibitors, angiotensin II receptor blockers and thiazide diuretics. These medications have a low rate of side effects, and they help protect your kidneys and heart, which are at high risk of damage from both diseases.

Watch your cholesterol

High levels of cholesterol and triglycerides increase your risk of heart attack and stroke. A healthy lifestyle is critically important. Focus on reducing your intake of saturated fats, trans fats and cholesterol and getting regular physical activity. Cholesterol recommendations for people with diabetes are generally as follows:

▶ Low-density lipoprotein (LDL, or the "bad") cholesterol less than 100 mg/dL of blood
▶ High-density lipoprotein (HDL, or "good") cholesterol higher than 40 mg/dL for men and 50 mg/dL for women
▶ Triglycerides under 150 mg/dL

If you don't achieve your goals, your doctor may prescribe a cholesterol-lowering drug called a statin, especially if:

▶ You're older than age 40
▶ You're under age 40 and you have other risk factors for cardiovascular disease
▶ You have cardiovascular disease

Studies, including the Heart Protection Study, suggest that taking statins can lower the risk of heart attack or stroke in people with diabetes even if they have normal cholesterol levels. Statin therapy isn't recommended for women who are pregnant.

If you have or are at significant risk of cardiovascular complications, research also suggests that taking an aspirin every day can greatly reduce the risk of heart attacks and other cardiovascular complications in people older than age 40 who have type 1 or 2 diabetes. Ask your doctor if aspirin therapy would be of benefit to you. A daily aspirin isn't recommended if you have liver disease.

Caring for your eyes

Diabetes is the leading cause of new cases of blindness in people ages 20 to 74. The American Diabetes Association (ADA) recommends an initial comprehensive eye exam by an eye specialist (ophthalmologist or optometrist) shortly after diagnosis if you have type 2 diabetes and within five years after onset if you have type 1 diabetes. After that, have an eye exam by a specialist yearly — or more often if you have eye damage (retinopathy) that's getting worse.

If your diabetes is poorly controlled, you have high blood pressure or kidney disease, or you're pregnant, you may need to see an eye specialist more than once a year. If your eyes are normal after an exam and your blood sugar (glucose) is under control, your eye specialist may recommend an eye exam every two to three years.

Don't wait for vision problems to develop before you see an eye specialist. Typically, by the time symptoms emerge, some permanent damage has already occurred.

Choose an eye specialist who has expertise and experience in diabetic retinopathy. Make sure this person knows you have diabetes and performs a thorough exam, including dilation of your pupils. Your eye exam may include a number of tests.

Visual acuity test
This test determines your level of vision and need for corrective lenses, and it establishes a baseline measurement for future eye exams.

External eye exam
An external eye exam measures your eye movements, along with the size of your pupils and their ability to respond to light.

Retinal exam
When doing a retinal exam, your eye specialist places medicated eyedrops into your eyes to dilate your pupils and check for damage to your retinas and the tiny blood vessels that nourish them. This is an especially important test for people with diabetes because retinal damage is the most common eye complication of diabetes.

Glaucoma test
A glaucoma test (tonometry) measures the pressure inside your eyes. Abnormally high pressure is an indicator of glaucoma — a disease that can gradually narrow your field of vision and produce tunnel vision and blindness. Diabetes increases your risk of developing glaucoma.

Slit-lamp exam
During a slit-lamp exam, your eye specialist evaluates the structures of your eyes, such as the cornea and iris. He or she also looks for cataracts, which cloud your lenses and can make you feel as if you're looking through wax paper or a smudgy window. Diabetes can spur cataracts to develop sooner than they otherwise would.

Eye photography
If you have eye damage or suspected damage, your eye specialist may take photos with specially designed cameras. These photos are meant to document the status of your vision and establish a baseline for future exams.

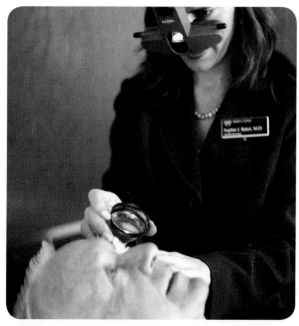

In this form of retinal examination, you lie back while the doctor holds your eye open and examines it with a bright light mounted on his or her forehead.

Caring for your feet

Diabetes can cause two potentially dangerous threats to your feet: It can damage the nerves in your feet, and it can reduce blood flow to your feet.

When the network of nerves in your feet is damaged, the sensation of pain in your feet is reduced. Because of this, you can develop a blister or cut your foot without realizing it.

Diabetes can also narrow your arteries, reducing blood flow to your feet. With less blood to nourish tissues in your feet, it's harder for sores to heal. An unnoticed cut or sore hidden beneath your socks and shoes can quickly develop into a larger problem.

Check your feet every day

Use your eyes and hands to examine your feet regularly. If you aren't able to see some parts of your feet, use a mirror or ask a family member or a friend to examine those locations.

Look for these common ailments:

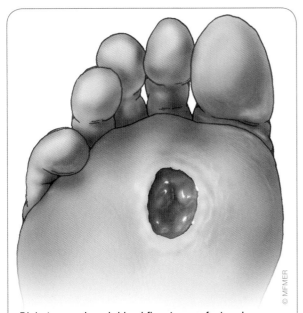

Diabetes can impair blood flow to your feet and cause nerve damage. Without proper attention and care, a small injury can develop into an open sore (ulcer) that can be difficult to treat.

- Blisters, cuts and bruises
- Cracking, peeling and wrinkling
- Redness, red streaks and swelling
- Feet that are pinker, paler, darker or redder than usual

Keep your feet clean and dry

Wash your feet each day with lukewarm water. To avoid burning your feet, test the water temperature with a thermometer. It should be no warmer than 90 F (32 C). Or test the water by touching a dampened washcloth to a sensitive area of your body, such as your face, neck or wrist.

Wash your feet with a gentle, massage-like motion, using a soft washcloth or sponge and a mild soap. Dry your skin by blotting or patting. Don't rub because you may accidentally damage your skin. Dry carefully between your toes to help prevent fungal infection.

Moisturize your skin

When diabetes damages your nerves, you may sweat less than normal, leaving your skin dry, especially on your feet. Dry skin can itch and crack, increasing your risk of an infection.

Keep the blood flowing

To help keep blood flowing to your feet, put your feet up when sitting, then move your ankles and toes frequently. Don't cross your legs for long, and don't wear tight socks.

Wear clean, dry socks

Wear socks made of fibers that pull (wick) sweat away from your skin, such as cotton and special acrylic fibers — not nylon. Avoid those with tight elastic bands that reduce circulation or that are thick or bulky. Bulky socks often fit poorly, and a poor fit can irritate your skin.

It's also a good idea to avoid mended socks with thick seams that can rub and irritate your skin. Among people with diabetes such socks can cause pressure sores.

Trim your toenails carefully

Cut your toenails straight across so that they're even with the end of your toe. File rough edges so that you don't have any sharp areas that could cut the neighboring toe. Be especially careful not to injure the surrounding skin. If you notice redness around the nails, report this to your doctor or your podiatrist.

Use foot products cautiously

Don't use a file or scissors on calluses, corns or bunions. You can injure your feet that way. Also, don't put chemicals on your feet, such as wart removers. See your doctor or podiatrist for problem calluses, corns, bunions or warts.

Wear shoes that protect your feet from injury

To help protect your feet and toes, follow these tips:

Protect against heat and cold
Don't use heating pads on your feet. Use proper footwear to avoid hot pavement in hot weather and to avoid frostbite in cold weather.

Always wear shoes
Wear slippers with soles around the house.

Check your shoes

Look inside your shoes for tears or rough edges that might injure your feet. Shake out your shoes before you put them on to make sure that nothing is inside, such as a pebble.

Select a comfortable and safe style of shoe
Good shoe design includes the following:

- **Soft leather tops.** Leather adapts to the shape of your foot and lets air circulate. Good air circulation is important because it reduces sweating, a major cause of skin irritation.
- **Closed-toe design.** Shoes with closed toes provide the best protection from cuts and scrapes.
- **Low-heeled shoes.** These shoes are safer, more comfortable and less damaging to your feet.
- **Flexible soles made from crepe or foam rubber.** These soles are the most comfortable for daily wear. They also act as good shock absorbers. The soles of your shoes should provide solid footing and not be slippery.

Have at least two pairs of shoes so that you can switch shoes each day. This gives your shoes time to completely dry out and regain their shape after each use. Don't wear wet shoes because moisture can shrink the material and make your shoes rub against your feet.

Seeing a podiatrist

Because foot care is especially important to people with diabetes, your primary care doctor or diabetes specialist may recommend a doctor who specializes in foot care (podiatrist). A podiatrist can teach you how to trim your toenails properly. If you have vision problems or significant loss of sensation in your feet, he or she can trim them for you.

A podiatrist can also teach you how to buy properly fitted shoes and prevent problems such as corns and calluses. If problems do occur, a podiatrist can help treat them to prevent more-serious conditions from developing. Even small sores can quickly turn into serious problems without proper treatment.

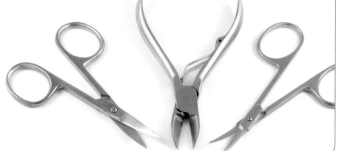

Does the shoe fit?

When you buy new shoes:

▶ Make sure the tip of each shoe extends at least a ¼ inch beyond your longest toe. The shoe tip also should be wide and long enough that your toes aren't cramped. Walk around the store with both of the new shoes on.

▶ If possible, try on shoes in early afternoon. Feet swell as the day goes on. If you buy shoes in the morning, they may feel too tight later on. Getting fitted at the end of the day may give you a fit that's too roomy in the morning.

▶ If one foot is bigger than the other, buy shoes to fit your larger foot.

▶ If you have reduced sensation in your feet, take the shoes home and wear them for 30 minutes. Then remove them and examine your feet. Red areas indicate pressure and a poor fit. If you see any red areas, return the shoes. If no problems occur, gradually increase the time you wear them by a half-hour to one hour each day.

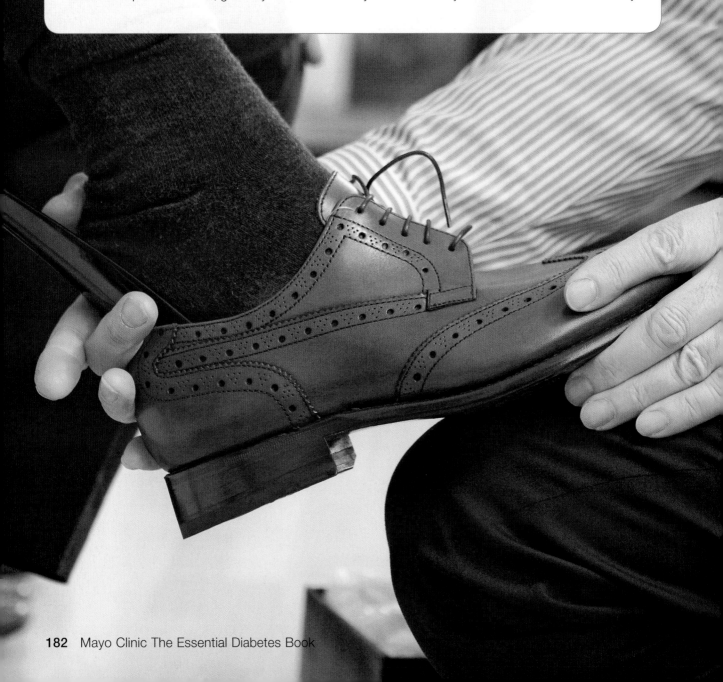

Caring for your teeth

High blood sugar (glucose) can impair your immune system, making it difficult to fight off bacteria and viruses that cause infection.

One common site of infection is your gums. That's because your mouth harbors many bacteria. If these germs settle in your gums and cause an infection, you may end up with gum disease that can cause your teeth to loosen and fall out.

In addition, limited research suggests that people with gum infections may be at increased risk of cardiovascular disease. One theory is that bacteria from the mouth gets into the bloodstream and may cause inflammation throughout the body, including the arteries. This may be linked with the development of artery-clogging plaques, possibly increasing the risk of a heart attack or stroke.

To help prevent damage to your gums and teeth:

▶ See your dentist twice a year for professional cleanings, and make sure your dentist knows that you have diabetes.
▶ Brush your teeth twice a day, using a soft nylon toothbrush, and brush the upper surface of your tongue.
▶ Floss daily. It helps remove plaque between your teeth and under your gumline.
▶ Look for early signs of gum disease, such as bleeding gums, redness and swelling. If you notice them, see your dentist.

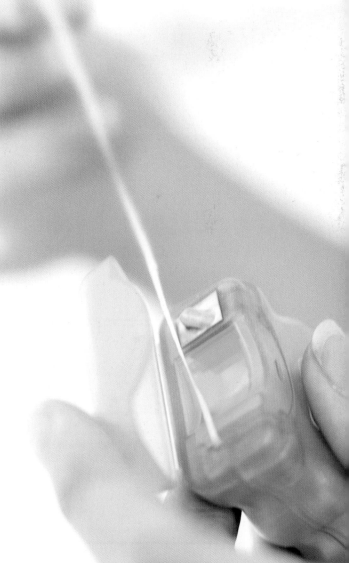

Don't smoke

People with diabetes who smoke are at least twice as likely as nonsmokers with diabetes to die of cardiovascular disease, such as heart attack or stroke. People with diabetes who smoke are also more likely to develop circulation problems in their feet.

Consider these risks:

▶ Smoking increases your risk of nerve damage and kidney disease.
▶ Smoking narrows and hardens your arteries. This increases your risk of heart attack and stroke and reduces blood flow to your legs, making it more difficult for wounds to heal.
▶ Smoking appears to impair your immune system, producing more colds and respiratory infections.

If you have diabetes and smoke, talk to your doctor about methods to quit. And don't be discouraged if your first attempts aren't successful. Stopping smoking can take several attempts, but it's vitally important to your health.

Getting vaccinated

Because high blood glucose can weaken your immune system, you may be more prone to complications from the flu (influenza) and pneumonia than are people who don't have diabetes. And if you have heart or kidney disease, you're at even higher risk of problems.

Annual flu shot

The best way to avoid the flu (influenza) or to reduce its symptoms is to have an annual flu shot (vaccination). In the United States, the best time to be vaccinated is in October or November. This allows your immunity to peak during the height of the flu season, which is generally December through March.

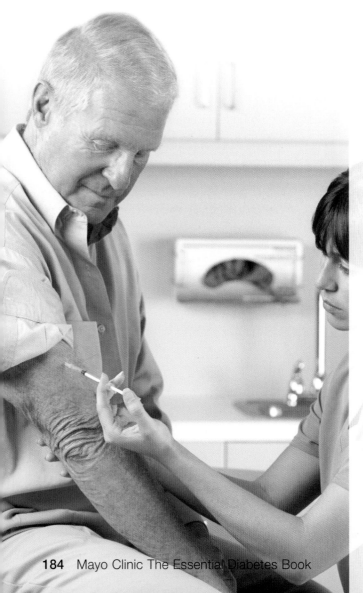

In other parts of the world, the flu season varies: In the Southern Hemisphere, it's primarily from April to September, and in the tropics, you can catch the flu year-round. So take this into account if you're traveling and get advice from your doctor or a travel medicine specialist.

In the U.S., flu shots are modified annually to protect you against those flu strains most likely to circulate during the coming winter.

The injectable vaccine contains only noninfectious viruses and can't cause the flu. (Special circumstances need to be considered when taking the intranasal vaccine.) The most common side effect is a little soreness at the spot where the injection is given. Ask your doctor if there are any other risks in your case.

Pneumonia vaccine

Most doctors recommend that people with diabetes receive the pneumonia (pneumococcal) vaccine. For healthy people age 65 or older, generally just one lifetime dose is recommended unless they were younger than 65 when first vaccinated.

However, a one-time booster after five years is often recommended if you have diabetes, renal failure or kidney transplantation. Check with your doctor for advice.

The pneumonia vaccine contains substances that activate your immune system (antigens). These antigens protect you against 85 to 90 percent of all forms of pneumonia found in the United States. Side effects of the pneumococcal vaccine are generally minor and include mild soreness or swelling at the injection site.

Other vaccinations

Make sure you're up to date on other important vaccinations, such as a tetanus shot and a booster shot every 10 years. Ask your doctor about getting vaccinated for protection against hepatitis B if you receive hemodialysis.

Managing stress

When you're under a lot of stress, it becomes more difficult to take good care of yourself and your diabetes. You might not eat well. You may not exercise. And you may not take your medication as prescribed. Excessive or prolonged stress also can increase production of hormones that block the effect of insulin, causing your blood sugar (glucose) to rise.

Stop and think about what causes you stress. Then ask yourself if you can do anything to change the situation. If a hectic day of running from one event to another causes stress, reduce your daily commitments. If certain friends or family members cause you stress, limit the time you spend with them. If your job is stressful, look for ways to help lighten the load, such as handing over some of your responsibilities to others. Also ask your health care team for advice.

The stress response

Stress is your response to an event — not the event itself. Often referred to as the fight-or-flight reaction, the stress response occurs automatically when you feel threatened. The threat can be any situation that is perceived — even falsely — as dangerous, so your perception is a key issue.

When you perceive a threat, your body responds by sending out a flood of hormones, including adrenaline and cortisol, into your bloodstream.

These hormones help focus your concentration, speed your reaction time, and increase your strength and agility. At the same time, your heart rate and blood pressure increase as more blood is pumped through your body, prepping you to do what's required to adapt and survive. This is called your stress response.

Not all stress is bad. Stress can be positive when it results in energy directed toward growth, action and change. This is the type of stress associated with the welcome birth of a child or a job promotion, for example. However, when you have too much stress, it lasts too long or it's linked with negative experiences, stress can be harmful to your health.

Individual reactions to stress

Your reaction to a stressful event may be different from someone else's. Some people are naturally laidback about most things, while others react strongly to the slightest hint of stress. Most people fall somewhere between those extremes.

Genetic variations may partly explain the differences. The genes that control the stress response keep most people on a fairly even keel, only occasionally priming the body for fight or flight. Overactive or underactive stress responses may stem from slight differences in these genes.

Life experiences may increase your sensitivity to stress as well. Strong stress reactions sometimes can be traced to early environmental factors. People who were exposed to extreme stress as children tend to be particularly vulnerable to stress as adults.

Learning to relax

Is it difficult for you to relax? Are you on the go all the time? Take steps to learn how to relax.

Relaxed breathing

Have you ever noticed how you breathe when you're stressed? Stress typically causes rapid, shallow breathing, which sustains other aspects of the stress response, such as a rapid heart rate. If you can get control of your breathing, the spiraling effects of acute stress will automatically decrease.

Practice relaxed breathing (also called deep breathing or diaphragmatic breathing) at least twice a day and whenever you begin to feel tense:

▶ **Inhale.** With your mouth closed and your shoulders relaxed, inhale slowly and deeply through your nose to the count of six. Allow the air to fill the muscle between your abdomen and your chest (diaphragm).
▶ Pause for a second.
▶ **Exhale.** Slowly release the air through your mouth as you count to six.
▶ Pause for a second.
▶ **Repeat.** Complete this breathing cycle several times.

You're breathing correctly when your abdomen — not your chest — moves with each breath. If you're lying down, place a paperback book on your abdomen. When you breathe in, the book should rise. When you breathe out, the book should go down.

Progressive muscle relaxation

Progressive muscle relaxation can reduce muscle tension. First, find a quiet place where you'll be free from interruption. Loosen tight clothing and remove your glasses or contacts if you'd like.

Tense each muscle group for at least five seconds, and then relax for up to 30 seconds. Repeat before moving to the next muscle group:

- **Upper part of your face.** Lift your eyebrows toward the ceiling, feeling the tension in your forehead and scalp. Relax. Repeat.
- **Central part of your face.** Squint your eyes tightly and wrinkle your nose and mouth, feeling the tension in the center of your face. Relax. Repeat.
- **Lower part of your face.** Gently clench your teeth and pull back the corners of your mouth toward your ears. Show your teeth like a snarling dog. Relax. Repeat.
- **Neck.** Gently touch your chin to your chest. Feel the pull in the back of your neck. Relax. Repeat.
- **Shoulders.** Pull your shoulders up toward your ears, feeling the tension in your shoulders, head, neck and upper back. Relax. Repeat.
- **Upper arms.** Pull your arms back and press your elbows in toward the sides of your body. Try not to tense your lower arms. Feel the tension in your arms, shoulders and into your back. Relax. Repeat.
- **Hands and lower arms.** Make a tight fist and pull up your wrists. Feel the tension in your hands, knuckles and lower arms. Relax. Repeat.
- **Chest, shoulders and upper back.** Pull your shoulders back as if you're trying to make your shoulder blades touch. Relax. Repeat.
- **Stomach.** Pull your stomach in toward your spine, tightening your abdominal muscles. Relax. Repeat.
- **Upper legs.** Squeeze your knees together. Feel the tension in your thighs. Relax. Repeat.
- **Lower legs.** Bend your ankles so that your toes point toward your face. Feel the tension in the front of your lower legs. Relax. Repeat.
- **Feet.** Turn your feet inward and curl your toes up and out. Relax. Repeat.

Perform progressive muscle relaxation at least once or twice each day for maximum benefit. Each session should last about 10 minutes. Your ability to relax will improve with practice. Be patient — eventually you can experience a greater sense of calm.

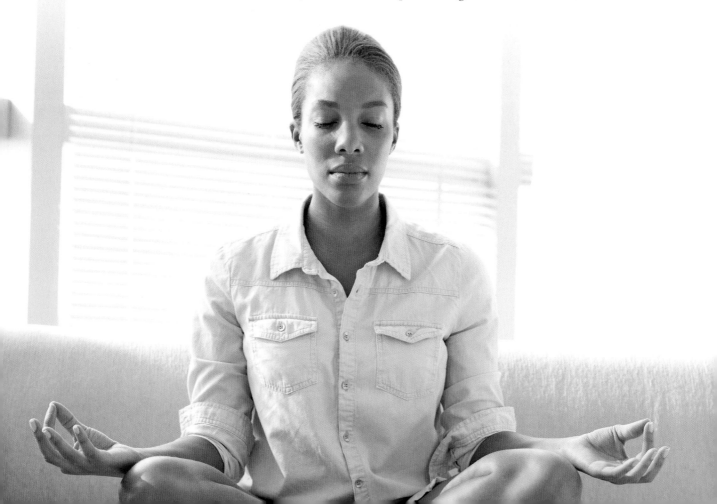

Listen and visualize

If you have about 10 minutes and a quiet room, you can take a mental vacation almost anytime. Consider listening to relaxation CDs or podcasts to help you unwind and rest your mind.

Options include:

▶ **Spoken word.** These recordings use spoken suggestions to guide your meditation, educate you on stress reduction or take you on an imaginary visual journey to a peaceful place.

▶ **Soothing music or nature sounds.** Music has the power to affect your thoughts and feelings. Soft, soothing music can help you relax and lower your stress level.

No one recording works for everyone, so try several to find which works best for you. Listen to samples in the store or online, or ask your friends or a stress management professional for recommendations.

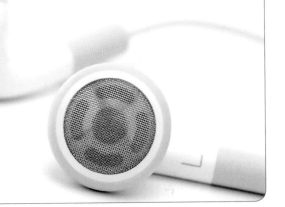

Meditation

Different types of meditation techniques can calm your mind and reduce your stress level.

Concentration meditation involves focusing your attention on one thing, such as your breathing, an image you visualize or a real image you look at — for example, a candle flame.

Here's a simple meditation technique:

▶ Put on comfortable clothes.
▶ Choose a quiet space where you won't be interrupted.
▶ Sit comfortably.
▶ Close your eyes, relax your muscles, and breathe slowly and naturally.
▶ For several minutes, slowly repeat a focus phrase (silently or aloud), such as "I am calm" or "I am serene." When other thoughts intrude, bring your attention back to your focus phrase.
▶ When you're finished, sit quietly for a minute or two to make the transition back to your normal routine.

The best-known example of meditation is prayer. You can pray using your own words, or you can read prayers written by others.

Meditation may be practiced on its own or as part of another relaxation therapy, such as yoga or tai chi.

Other relaxation techniques

You can choose many other relaxation techniques, such as:

▶ **Tai chi.** Tai chi (TIE-CHEE) involves slow, gentle, dance-like movements. Each movement or posture flows into the next without pausing. Tai chi can reduce stress and improve balance and flexibility. This form of exercise is generally safe for people of all ages and levels of fitness because the low-impact movements put minimal stress on muscles and joints.

▶ **Yoga.** Yoga typically combines gentle breathing exercises with precise movements through a series of postures. For some people, yoga is a spiritual path. For others, yoga is a way to promote physical flexibility, strength and endurance. In either case, yoga may help you to relax and manage stress. Although yoga is generally safe, some yoga positions can put a strain on your lower back and joints.

▶ **Massage.** Massage is the kneading, stroking and manipulation of your body's soft tissues — your skin, muscles and tendons. It may be used to relieve muscle tension or promote relaxation as people undergo other types of medical treatment. For healthy people, it can be a simple stress reliever. Massage is generally safe as long as a trained therapist does it.

Keeping your cool

You can help keep your cool and lighten your load by remembering the four A's to managing stress: Avoid, alter, adapt or accept.

Avoid

A lot of needless stress can simply be avoided:

▶ **Take control of your surroundings.** Does rush-hour traffic drive you crazy? Plan to leave earlier for work. Hate waiting in line at the corporate cafeteria? Pack your own lunch.

▶ **Avoid contact with someone who bothers you.** If you have a co-worker who causes your jaw to tense, put physical distance between you and this person.

▶ **Learn to say no.** You have a lot of responsibilities and demands on your time. Turn down requests that drain your energy and that aren't essential.

Alter

Attempt to change your situation, so things work better in the future:

▶ **Respectfully ask others to change their behavior and be willing to do the same.** Small problems often create larger ones when they aren't resolved.

▶ **Communicate your feelings openly.** Use "I" statements, as in "I feel frustrated by a heavier workload. Is there something we can do to balance things out?"

▶ **Take risks.** Sometimes inaction creates tension. Vie for the assignment you really want at work. Taking a chance may feel good, regardless of the outcome.

Adapt

Adapting — changing your standards or expectations — is one of the best ways to deal with stress:

▶ **Adjust your standards.** Do you need to vacuum and dust twice a week, or can you accept less often — especially on busy weeks? Redefine cleanliness, success and perfection.

▶ **Practice thought stopping.** Stop gloomy thoughts immediately. Refuse to replay a stressful situation as negative, and it may cease to be so.

▶ **Use humor.** Allow yourself to see an terrible day as comical. Laugh at the lunacy of it all.

Accept

If you have no choice but to accept things as they are, try to:

▶ **Talk with someone.** Phone a friend or schedule a coffee break. You'll feel better after talking it out.

▶ **Forgive.** It takes energy to be angry. Forgiving may take practice, but by doing so, you'll free yourself from burning more negative energy.

▶ **Smile.** It may improve your mood. Smiles are contagious. Before long, you're likely to see your smile sincerely reflected back at you.

Making time for yourself

Do you take time to focus on yourself and do things that you enjoy? Some people are so involved in their work that they don't know the first thing about leisure. And that's too bad, because leisure activities can reduce your stress and improve your outlook on life.

Not taking time for yourself can affect personal relationships and decrease your effectiveness and enthusiasm for your roles at work and home.

Find leisure activities to meet your needs

Leisure activities — what you choose to do during your free time — vary from person to person. What someone else finds interesting and pleasurable may be incredibly boring for you. But if you've been burying your nose in your work, you may not even know what you want to do for leisure.

One approach is to look at your self-care needs:

▶ **Are you getting enough physical activity and exercise?** Regular physical activity promotes both physical and mental health.

▶ **Do you get enough rest and relaxation?** Try to get enough sleep and consider doing restful activities (such as reading, listening to music or meditating) to help you balance an active day.

- **Do you challenge yourself mentally?** Keep your mind active with crossword puzzles, word games, writing, a class or anything else that's mentally stimulating.
- **Are you meeting your spiritual needs?** Depending on how you define spirituality, participate in organized religious activities, experience the beauty of nature, or express yourself in music, meditation or art.
- **Do you have enough social contact with others?** Consider dining out with friends, having friends over, or joining a musical group or a sports league.
- **Do you have enough alone time?** Solitary time lets you focus on your inner thoughts and take a break from meeting the demands of others. Read a book, write in a journal, meditate or do anything that appeals to you.
- **Are you using your creative abilities?** Dance, write, paint, cook, play an instrument — do anything that gets your creative juices flowing.
- **Are you interested in service to others?** You might do volunteer work for an agency or community project, cook or do yardwork for a neighbor, or care for a friend's child.
- **Is there novelty or adventure in your life?** Experience new things. Consider traveling, hiking, camping, or learning a new skill or hobby.

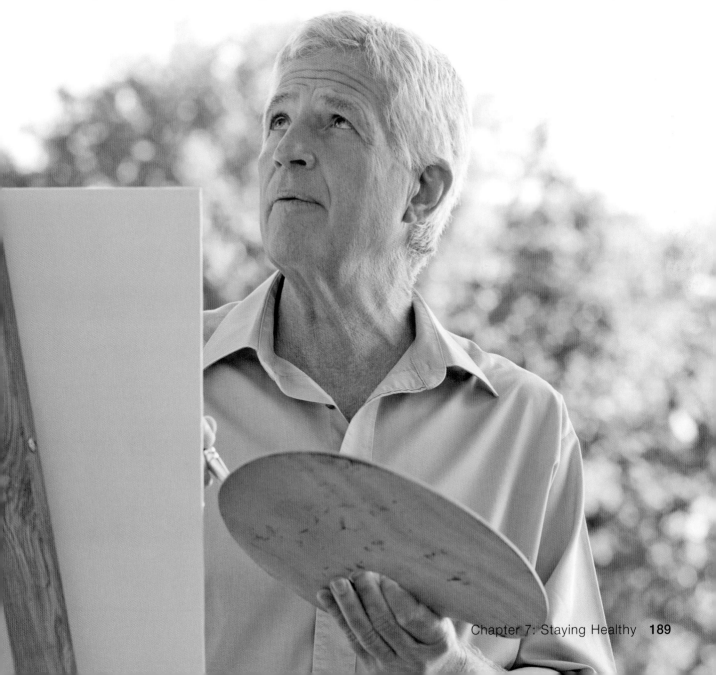

Preparing for pregnancy

You have diabetes and are thinking about becoming pregnant. You look forward to becoming a mother and want to give birth to a healthy baby.

Ready for some good news? Women with diabetes who control their blood sugar (glucose) before they're pregnant and during their pregnancy have almost the same chance of having a healthy baby as do women without diabetes. Your blood glucose level should be in good control for three to six months before you try to get pregnant.

Why it's best to plan your pregnancy

To prevent diabetes-related complications, make sure your blood glucose is under control before you become pregnant. Your blood glucose not only affects your health, it affects your baby's health.

Your baby's organs form during the first six to eight weeks of pregnancy. But you probably won't know you're pregnant until your baby has been growing for two to four weeks. So if you don't plan your pregnancy and you have poor blood glucose control, your baby's risk of birth defects is much higher.

Birth defects can affect your baby's brain, heart and kidneys. To help prevent birth defects, your doctor will recommend that you take a multivitamin with folic acid each day, ideally starting three months before you get pregnant, and a prenatal vitamin throughout your pregnancy.

When you become pregnant

Like most women, you're probably experiencing the joys and fears of having a baby. But you're concerned about the effects diabetes can have on your body, on labor and on delivery, and you're concerned about the health of your baby.

Because of your diabetes, you'll have extra challenges to deal with during your pregnancy. But the most important challenge is keeping your blood glu-

Tight control reduces birth defects

Blood glucose control is crucial not only to your health but also to the health of your unborn child. If during the first six to eight weeks of your baby's development — when your baby's heart, lungs, kidneys and brain are being formed — your blood glucose is too high, your baby is at increased risk of birth defects. A high level of ketones in your blood (diabetic ketoacidosis) also can cause miscarriage. Later in pregnancy, uncontrolled blood glucose can lead to premature birth or stillbirth or other problems. Fortunately, most of these problems are preventable or treatable.

cose under tight control. With the help of your health care team, you can monitor your blood glucose and avoid complications as your pregnancy progresses.

In addition to the health care team members listed on page 172, your team may include:

▶ An obstetrician with special training in handling high-risk pregnancies and pregnancies of women with diabetes.
▶ A pediatrician or neonatologist with expertise in treating babies born to women with diabetes. (A pediatrician specializes in the treatment of children, and a neonatologist is a pediatrician who specializes in the care of sick newborn babies.)

If you live in a small town or a rural area and don't have easy access to specialists, ask your doctor about his or her experience treating pregnant women with diabetes. Find out if this doctor has access to a specialist at a nearby university or metropolitan area. Your doctor may have you visit a specialist once during your pregnancy and consult with the specialist during your pregnancy.

Tight control

As in the pre-pregnancy stage, during your pregnancy your chief goal is to keep your blood glucose under tight control. Your doctor will tell you what your target blood glucose range is.

If you have type 2 diabetes, you may stop taking oral medications and take insulin to manage your blood glucose while you're pregnant. One reason is that intensive insulin therapy can achieve tighter control of your blood glucose. Another is that the safety of oral diabetes medications for pregnant women and unborn babies is unknown when taken during all nine months of pregnancy.

If you need to switch to insulin therapy, your health care team will teach you how to take insulin. The team will also tell you how often to check your blood glucose.

What to expect during pregnancy

Here's what can happen as your pregnancy progresses.

First trimester

During the first 10 to 12 weeks of your pregnancy, you'll probably see your obstetrician fairly frequently. This is the time that your baby's organs are developing, so your blood glucose needs to be as close to normal as possible to prevent birth defects. Frequent blood glucose monitoring can help you do this.

Because your need for insulin may drop slightly during this time, be alert to signs of low blood glucose. If morning sickness makes you miserable, talk with your doctor about medication to treat nausea.

Second trimester

The second trimester is when you'll likely receive an ultrasound to check the health of your baby. Your doctor also will keep track of your weight gain.

If your weight is normal when you start your pregnancy, research suggests a total gain of 25 to 35 pounds is healthiest for you and your baby. If you're too thin, you may need to gain more. If you're obese, you may need to work with a dietitian to limit your weight gain.

If you take insulin, expect your insulin requirements to rise gradually to about week 20 and then accelerate dramatically. Hormones made by the placenta to help your baby grow block the effect of your insulin, so you'll need significantly more to compensate.

At this stage of your pregnancy, it's also important to see an eye specialist. Damage to the small blood vessels in your eyes can progress during pregnancy.

Third trimester

During the final three months of your pregnancy, you'll need careful monitoring. Your doctor will check for complications that can occur during the late stage of any pregnancy, such as high blood pressure (hypertension), swollen ankles from fluid buildup and kidney problems. Your doctor may also recommend that you have your eyes examined again to check for eye damage.

Because women with diabetes are more likely to give birth to babies who weigh more than 9 pounds, you may receive another ultrasound to assess the size and health of your baby. At this stage, any potential problem for you or your baby may prompt early delivery.

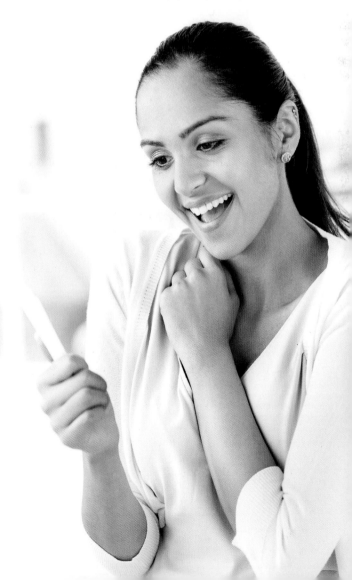

Labor and delivery

Your health care team will help you determine the best time and safest method to deliver your baby. Delivering your baby at home with a nurse-midwife generally isn't recommended because of the increased potential for problems due to your diabetes.

As long as your blood glucose remains under control, and you and your baby don't experience complications, you can expect a normal vaginal delivery.

During labor, your blood glucose will be closely monitored to prevent a large decrease or increase in your glucose levels. Because your body is working so hard and using glucose as energy, you'll likely need less insulin.

If there are complications or your baby is too large for a safe vaginal delivery, your baby may be delivered by cesarean section through an incision in your lower abdominal and uterine walls. Regardless of the delivery method, the result for most women who've maintained good blood glucose control is a healthy baby.

Following delivery, your insulin needs will decrease. However, it may take weeks to months before your body changes are complete and you return to your normal medication regimen.

Gestational diabetes

Gestational diabetes only occurs during the time you're pregnant, generally developing in the second or third trimester. Like other forms of diabetes, gestational diabetes causes your blood glucose to become too high. If untreated or uncontrolled, gestational diabetes can result in health problems for both you and your baby.

During pregnancy, your placenta — the organ that supplies your baby with nutrients through the umbilical cord — produces hormones that prevent insulin from doing its job. These hormones are vital to preserving your pregnancy. Yet they also make your cells more resistant to insulin. As your placenta grows larger in the second and third trimesters, it secretes even more of these hormones, further increasing insulin resistance.

Normally, your pancreas responds by producing enough extra insulin to overcome this resistance. But you may need up to three times as much insulin as normal, and sometimes your pancreas simply can't keep up. When this happens, too little glucose gets into your cells and too much stays in your blood.

Gestational diabetes usually occurs about the 20th to 24th week of pregnancy, and testing is usually recommended by the 24th to 28th week of pregnancy. After your baby is born and placental hormones disappear from your bloodstream, your blood glucose levels should quickly return to normal.

Most women don't experience any signs or symptoms of gestational diabetes. When they do occur, signs and symptoms may include excessive thirst and increased urination.

Risk factors

Any woman can develop gestational diabetes, but factors that increase your risk include:

- Age older than 25
- Family history of gestational diabetes
- Gestational diabetes in a previous pregnancy
- Being overweight before pregnancy
- Certain races, including African-American, Hispanic or American Indian (for reasons that aren't clear)
- Unexplained stillbirth
- Delivering a baby that weighs more than 9 pounds

Screening and diagnosis

In some places, screening for gestational diabetes is a routine part of prenatal care. To screen for gestational diabetes, most doctors recommend a glucose challenge test. This test is usually done between 24 and 28 weeks of pregnancy. However, if your doctor thinks you're at high risk, he or she may recommend that you have the test done earlier.

The glucose challenge test is a modified version of the oral glucose tolerance test, explained on page 21.

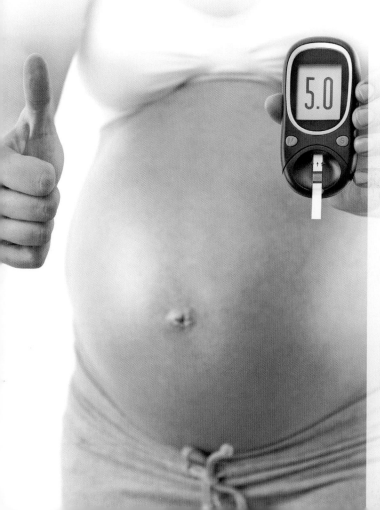

Typically, if you receive an abnormal result on the challenge test, your doctor will recommend follow-up glucose tolerance testing, which is done after an overnight fast.

Treatment

Controlling your blood glucose is essential to keeping your baby healthy and also avoiding dangerous complications for you both.

Monitoring your blood glucose is a key part of your treatment program to see if your blood sugar is staying within a normal range. Most women with gestational diabetes are able to control their blood glucose with diet and exercise, but some may also need insulin or other medications.

Results of a recent study support more-aggressive treatment in women with gestational diabetes. Researchers compared pregnancy outcomes in two groups. One group received aggressive treatment to maintain tight glucose control — dietary advice, more-frequent blood glucose monitoring and insulin injections for glucose levels above a desired range. The other group received routine care, glucose wasn't monitored as often, and they may or may not have used insulin.

The women who received aggressive treatment with insulin maintained tighter glucose control and developed significantly fewer childbirth problems than did the women under routine care. These results will likely affect future medical management of gestational diabetes.

In addition, a recent small study indicates that glyburide (Diabeta, Glynase), an oral drug, may be safe for women with gestational diabetes after the first trimester. There was no increase in complications.

After delivery

To make sure that your glucose level has returned to normal after your baby is born, you'll typically have your blood glucose checked often after delivery and again in six weeks. Once you've had gestational diabetes, continue to have your blood glucose tested at least once a year.

And remember: The very steps you're taking to control your blood glucose — such as eating a healthy diet and getting regular exercise — may also help prevent you from developing type 2 diabetes in the future.

Pregnancy complications from uncontrolled blood glucose

Most women with diabetes (any type) deliver healthy babies. However, untreated or uncontrolled blood glucose levels can cause serious problems.

Complications that may affect your baby

Keeping your blood glucose levels within a normal range can reduce the risk of complications, such as:

Macrosomia. Extra glucose can cross the placenta and end up in your baby's blood. When that happens, your baby's pancreas makes extra insulin to process the extra glucose, and this can cause your baby to grow too large (macrosomia).

Shoulder dystocia. If you have a very large baby, the shoulders may be too big to move through the birth canal, a potentially life-threatening emergency known as shoulder dystocia (dis-TOE-shuh). In most cases, doctors can perform maneuvers to free the baby.

Hypoglycemia. Sometimes, babies of mothers with diabetes develop low blood glucose (hypoglycemia) shortly after birth. That's because they've been receiving large amounts of blood glucose from their mothers, and their own insulin production is high. Hypoglycemia is easily detected and treated.

Respiratory distress syndrome. Babies born prematurely to mothers with diabetes are more likely to develop respiratory distress syndrome, a condition that makes breathing difficult.

Jaundice. Jaundice is a yellowish discoloration of the skin and the whites of the eyes from a buildup of old blood cells that aren't being cleared away fast enough by your baby's liver. This is easily treated, but requires careful monitoring.

Stillbirth or death. If the mother's diabetes goes undetected, a baby has an increased risk of stillbirth or death as a newborn.

Complications that may affect you

If you have diabetes, you may be at risk of:

Preeclampsia. A condition called preeclampsia (pree-uh-KLAMP-see-uh) is primarily characterized by a significant increase in blood pressure. Left untreated, it can lead to serious, even deadly complications for the mother and baby.

Having to have a C-section. Having diabetes isn't a reason to schedule a cesarean delivery, commonly called a C-section, but your doctor may recommend one if your baby has macrosomia.

Understanding menstruation and diabetes

Your ovaries produce the hormones estrogen and progesterone, which regulate your reproductive (menstrual) cycle. As the hormone levels fluctuate during the cycle, so can your blood glucose.

Most women who have menstruation-related changes in blood glucose notice it in the seven to 14 days before bleeding begins. Blood glucose generally stabilizes a day or two after the period starts. These changes tend to be more noticeable in women with premenstrual syndrome (PMS).

Premenstrual syndrome is a condition that occurs in some women about a week before menstruation. Symptoms include mood swings, tender breasts, bloating, lethargy, food cravings and lack of concentration. Giving in to cravings for carbohydrates and fats also can make blood glucose control more difficult.

High blood glucose can also lead to other problems, such as:

▶ Yeast infections of the vagina
▶ Irregular menstrual periods
▶ Loss of skin sensation around the vaginal area

What you can do

Keep a log. Record your blood glucose levels on a daily basis. Also jot down the day your period begins and the day that it ends.

Look for patterns in your blood glucose levels, especially the week before your period. Then talk with your doctor.

Your doctor may recommend changes in your medication dose or schedule, or your eating or exercise regimens, to make up for hormone-related swings in your blood glucose.

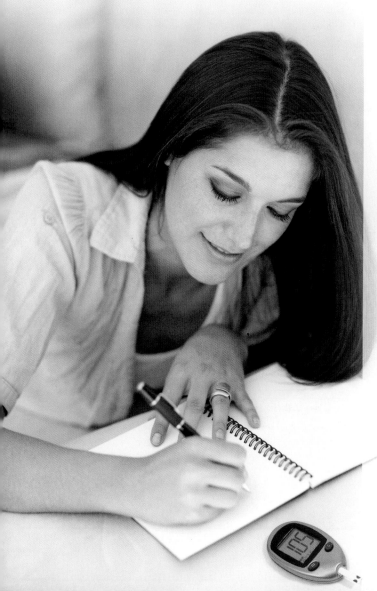

Dealing with menopause

Menopause — and the years leading up to it when your body gradually produces less estrogen and progesterone, called perimenopause — may present unique challenges if you have diabetes.

When 12 months have passed since your last period, you've reached menopause. Menopause most often occurs between the ages of 45 and 55, but it can occur at younger or older ages. As you approach menopause, your ovaries gradually stop producing the hormones estrogen and progesterone.

How these hormonal changes affect blood glucose varies, depending on the individual. Many women notice that their blood glucose levels are more variable (increases and decreases) and less predictable than before. Hormonal changes as well as swings in your blood glucose levels can contribute to menopausal symptoms such as mood changes, fatigue and hot flashes.

Similar symptoms

You may mistake menopausal symptoms such as hot flashes, moodiness and short-term memory loss for symptoms of low blood glucose. If you incorrectly assume these symptoms are due to low blood glucose, you may consume unnecessary calories to try to raise your blood glucose and cause it to go too high. The combination of menopause and diabetes can also cause other problems, such as:

▶ **Vaginal dryness.** Decreased blood flow to the vagina causes its lining to become thin and dry.
▶ **Yeast infections.** Increased levels of glucose in vaginal mucus and vaginal secretions that are less acidic and protective increase susceptibility to such infections.
▶ **Urinary tract infections.** Thinning of the lining of the bladder increases susceptibility to infections.

Although it's easy to confuse the symptoms of menopause and diabetes and to treat your diabetes inappropriately as a result, you can take steps to reduce such problems.

What you can do

There are key steps you can take to manage your diabetes during menopause.

Measure your blood glucose frequently

You may have to check your blood glucose three or four times a day, and occasionally during the night. Keeping a log of your levels and symptoms can help your doctor make necessary adjustments in your treatment.

Work with your doctor to adjust diabetes medications

If your blood glucose levels increase, you may need to increase the dosage of your diabetes medications or take a new medication.

This is especially likely if you gain weight or become less physically active. If your blood glucose decreases, you may need to reduce your dosages. Your need for insulin, for example, may significantly decline.

Ask your doctor if you need a cholesterol-lowering drug

If you have diabetes, you're at increased risk of heart and blood vessel (cardiovascular) disease. High levels of total and low-density lipoprotein (LDL or the "bad") cholesterol add to this risk, as does menopause.

As a result, many people with diabetes need a cholesterol-lowering medication — usually a statin — to reduce their risk of heart attack, stroke and other cardiovascular diseases.

Get help for menopausal symptoms

You may want to see a gynecologist or women's health specialist for help with especially bothersome symptoms, such as intense hot flashes or painful vaginal dryness and thinning.

If you're having problems with vaginal symptoms, for example, your doctor can prescribe treatments to help restore moisture. And antibiotics can help treat urinary tract infections. If weight gain is a problem — a concern for many women who reach menopause — consult with a dietitian to help review your meal plans.

Living with erectile dysfunction

It's estimated that more than half the men age 50 and older who have diabetes experience some degree of erectile dysfunction, sometimes called impotence. But few of them talk about it with their doctors. This is too bad because if they did, chances are good treatments — ranging from medications to surgery — could help restore sexual function for most.

Erectile dysfunction refers to the inability to achieve an erection of the penis or to maintain an erection long enough for sexual intercourse.

Causes

Male sexual arousal is a complex process involving the brain, hormones, emotions, nerves, muscles and blood vessels. If something affects any of these systems — or the delicate balance among them — erectile dysfunction can result.

Erectile dysfunction can result from physical or psychological factors. The most common causes in men with diabetes are physical problems due to poor blood glucose control or long-term effects of the disease.

Excess blood sugar (glucose) can damage the nerves and blood vessels responsible for erections, and not enough blood reaches the penis to cause an erection.

Psychological factors that can produce erectile dysfunction include stress, anxiety, fatigue or depression. They can interfere with your body's normal production of hormones and how your brain responds to them, preventing erections from occurring. Certain medications also can cause erectile dysfunction, including some drugs used to treat high blood pressure, anxiety and depression.

If you're experiencing erectile dysfunction, make sure your doctor is aware of all of the medications that you take.

When to seek medical advice

It's normal to experience erectile dysfunction on occasion. But if this problem lasts longer than two months or is recurring, see your doctor for a physical exam or for a referral to a doctor who specializes in erectile problems.

Several types of treatment are available. The cause and severity of your condition are important factors in determining the best treatment or combination of treatments for you. Don't try to combine medications or treatments on your own, and don't take more than the prescribed doses. Find out if your insurance may help cover the cost of treatment.

Oral drugs

Sildenafil (Viagra), tadalafil (Cialis, Adcirca) and vardenafil (Levitra, Staxyn) are phosphodiesterase (fos-foe-die-es-ter-ase) type 5 inhibitors, also called PDE5 inhibitors.

For some men with erectile dysfunction resulting from diabetes, these medications can improve sexual function, but they aren't effective for everyone. Unlike other treatments for erectile dysfunction, these drugs produce a more natural erection instead of an artificial one. They can help you respond to sexual or psychological stimulation by relaxing the smooth muscle tissue in the penis, which in turn increases blood flow in the penis and makes it easier for you to achieve and maintain an erection.

All of these drugs are taken about an hour before intercourse. The drugs are effective for varying lengths of time (from about four to 36 hours) and shouldn't be used more often than directed by your doctor.

Safety issues

Medications for erectile dysfunction aren't safe for all men. You shouldn't take these drugs if you're also taking nitrates, such as nitroglycerin.

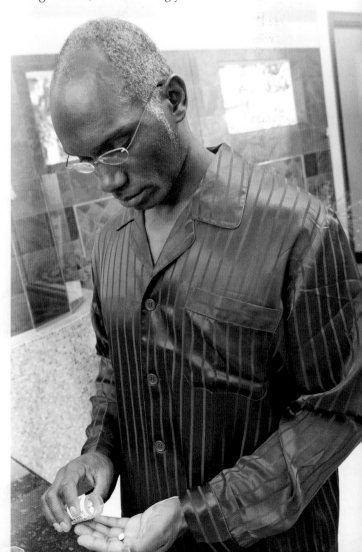

If these drugs are taken together with some blood pressure and prostate medications, this mix of medicine can substantially lower your blood pressure and produce a fatal heart attack.

This class of drugs can cause other side effects. The drugs may produce facial flushing, which generally lasts no more than five to 10 minutes. You may also experience a temporary mild headache or an upset stomach. Higher doses can produce short-term visual problems: a slight bluish tinge to objects, blurred vision and increased light sensitivity. These effects generally go away a few hours after taking the drug.

Specific instructions vary for each drug, so review the instructions with your doctor before taking.

Alprostadil

Alprostadil (al-PROS-tuh-dil) is a synthetic version of the chemical prostaglandin E1. As with oral drugs,

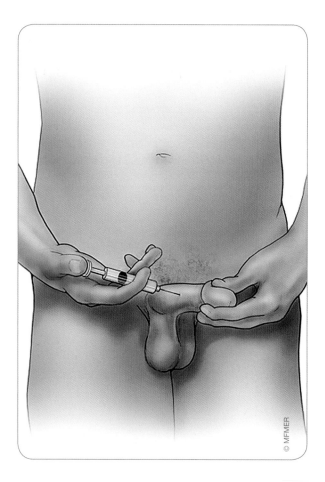

this medication helps relax smooth muscle tissue in the penis, which enhances the blood flow needed for an erection. There are two ways to use alprostadil: by self-administered intraurethral (in-truh-u-REE-thrul) therapy or self-injection therapy.

Self-administered intraurethral therapy

This method's trade name is Medicated Urethral System for Erection (MUSE).

It involves using a disposable applicator to insert a tiny suppository — about half the size of a grain of rice — into the tip of your penis. The suppository, placed about 2 inches into your urethra, is absorbed by erectile tissue in your penis, increasing the blood flow that causes an erection. Some men find this method to be uncomfortable.

Side effects may include pain, minor bleeding or burning in the urethra, or dizziness.

Self-injection therapy

With this method, you use a fine needle to inject alprostadil (Caverject Impulse, Edex) into the base or side of your penis. This generally produces an erection in five to 20 minutes that lasts about an hour.

Alprostadil injections are an effective treatment for many men with erectile dysfunction. Pain from the injection site is usually minor. Other side effects may include bleeding from the injection, prolonged erection or, rarely, formation of fibrous tissue at the injection site.

Injecting a mixture of alprostadil with either of the prescription drugs papaverine or phentolamine may be less expensive and more effective.

Vacuum devices

Some men turn to vacuum devices when medication is ineffective or its side effects are too bothersome. This treatment involves the use of an external vacuum and one or more rubber bands (tension rings).

You begin by placing a hollow plastic tube (available by prescription) over your penis. You then use a hand pump to create a vacuum in the tube and pull blood into your penis, producing an erection. You then slip off an elastic ring (mounted on the base of the plastic tube), pulling it around the base of your penis.

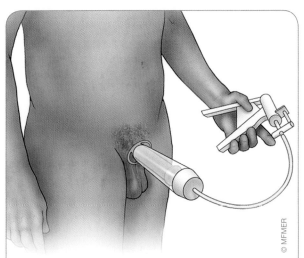

The vacuum device (shown above) has a hand pump to draw blood into the penis, creating an erection. An elastic ring placed at the base of the penis keeps it erect.

Self-injection therapy for erectile dysfunction (shown on the opposite page) involves injecting medication directly into a specific area of the penis to increase blood flow and cause an erection.

This traps the blood inside your penis, allowing you to keep your erection once the tube is removed.

You should remove the ring within 30 minutes to restore normal blood flow to your penis. If you don't, you could damage penile tissue.

Penile implants

If you've tried medication or a vacuum device and it hasn't worked or has been uncomfortable, you might consider a surgical implant. However, this type of treatment is often expensive, and as with any surgery, there is a small risk of complications, such as infection.

Semirigid, bendable rod

A semirigid, bendable rod type of implant is the easiest to use and the least likely to malfunction. Two hard but flexible rods made of wires and covered with silicone or polyurethane are placed inside your penis.

They give you a permanent erection. You bend your penis down toward your body to hide the erection and bend it up to have sexual intercourse.

Although it takes some getting used to, this implant requires less surgical time than other implants do, has no mechanical parts to break and has a high success rate.

Inflatable

These implants work more naturally than do the semirigid rods. Instead of having a permanent erection, you produce an erection only when you want one.

One version includes two hollow cylinders that are placed into your penis. These cylinders are connected to a tiny pump in your scrotum and to a reservoir in either your scrotum or your lower abdomen.

When you squeeze the pump, fluid from the reservoir fills the cylinders and produces an erection. The device is easily concealed and very effective, but it's more likely than other implants to have mechanical failure.

Another version doesn't involve a pump. Instead, a device near the head of your penis controls the flow of fluid inside the cylinders. To get an erection, you squeeze the head of your penis. This releases fluid into the cylinders. To shift the fluid back into place and produce a limp penis, you bend the implant and press a release valve.

Counseling

Erectile dysfunction typically causes anxiety, stress, misunderstanding and frustration to both partners. Psychological factors can play a significant role in this disorder and can be effectively treated with the aid of a psychiatrist, psychologist or other licensed therapist with experience in treating sexual problems.

Pursuing both the psychological and physical factors of erectile dysfunction is very important to a successful treatment outcome.

Chapter 8
If Your Child Has Diabetes

Type 1 diabetes 203

Type 2 diabetes 205

Caring for medical needs 208

Emotional and social issues 210

Good habits for staying healthy 212

Surviving sick days 215

A visit with Dr. Seema Kumar

"Type 2 diabetes, previously known as adult-onset diabetes, is becoming more common in children and adolescents. The epidemic of childhood obesity and the low level of physical activity among young people are major contributors to the increase in type 2 diabetes during childhood and adolescence."

The word *diabetes* comes from a Greek word meaning a "flowing through." It refers to the increased urine output seen in individuals with this condition. Diabetes is one of the most common chronic diseases in children and adolescents. About 215,000 people below the age of 20 have diabetes. Individuals with diabetes mellitus fall into two broad groups: those who have a deficiency of insulin (type 1) and those with a diminished effectiveness of insulin (type 2).

Type 1 diabetes accounts for the majority of diabetes seen during childhood in the United States and has a prevalence rate of 2 per 1,000 children between ages 0 and 19. Each year, more than 15,000 young people are diagnosed with type 1 diabetes. Type 2 diabetes begins when the body develops a resistance to insulin and no longer uses the insulin properly. As the need for insulin rises, the pancreas gradually loses its ability to produce sufficient amounts of insulin to regulate blood sugar (glucose). Type 2 diabetes, previously known as adult-onset diabetes, is becoming more common in children and adolescents. The epidemic of childhood obesity and the low level of physical activity among young people are major contributors to the increase in type 2 diabetes during childhood and adolescence. Those affected with type 2 diabetes belong to all ethnic groups, but it is more commonly seen in nonwhite groups such as black Americans, Native Americans and Mexican-Americans.

This chapter will discuss a number of issues related to juvenile diabetes, including the medical management of children with type 1 and type 2 diabetes mellitus. Since type 1 diabetes is characterized by insulin deficiency, all young people with this condition must take insulin delivered by injection or a pump. Treatment for type 1 diabetes is a lifelong commitment of

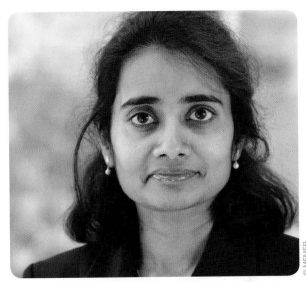

Seema Kumar, M.D.
Pediatric Endocrinology

monitoring blood sugar, taking insulin, maintaining a healthy weight, eating healthy foods and getting regular exercise.

Individuals with type 2 diabetes have insulin resistance and therefore lifestyle modifications consisting of a healthy diet, regular exercise and weight control are crucial in optimal management of these children. Medications also may be considered. Many medications that have been approved for treatment of type 2 diabetes in adults have not been used in children. Children and adolescents with type 2 diabetes who have significantly high blood glucose values at the time of diagnosis or who don't respond well to oral medications may need insulin for optimal management.

The long-term complications of diabetes result from the effects to blood vessels caused by elevated blood glucose levels. Keeping blood sugars close to normal can help prevent long-term complications of diabetes mellitus. Optimal blood glucose control helps promote normal growth and development during childhood. It's also needed to prevent the immediate dangers of blood glucose levels that are either too high or too low.

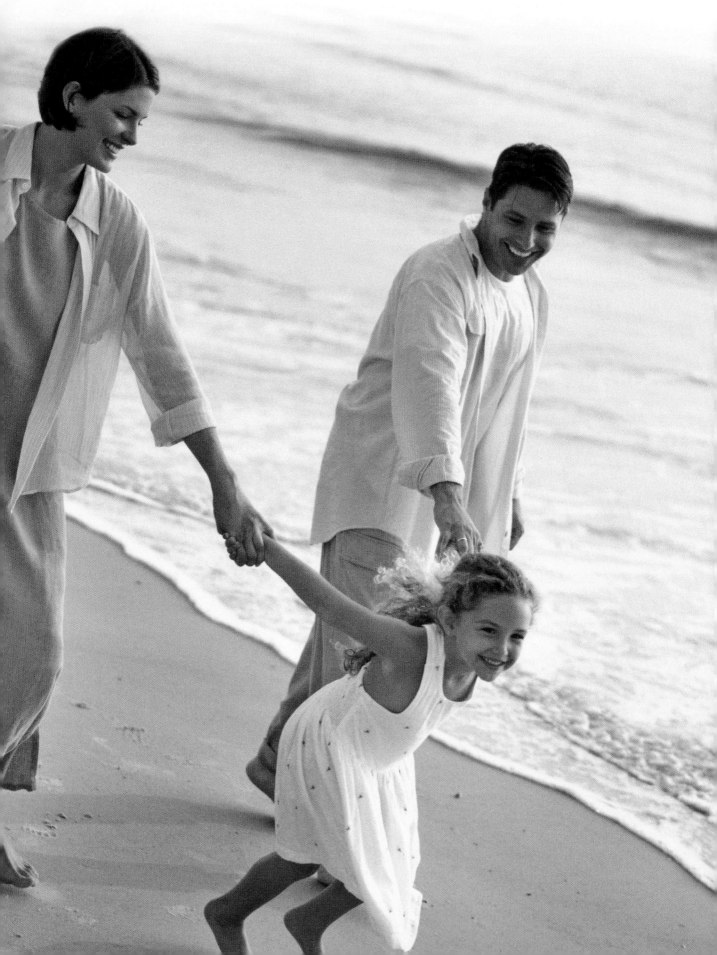

If your son or daughter was recently diagnosed with diabetes, chances are you've launched a frenzied mission to find out everything you can about managing this condition. If that's the case, take a step back and remind yourself that the last thing your child needs now is an exhausted, stressed-out parent.

It's important to learn as much as you can about diabetes and its management. As you gain knowledge, you'll also gain confidence that your child can still thrive with diabetes. However, it takes time to get a grasp on diabetes and to develop the best treatment plan for your child.

Your starting point will depend on whether your child has type 1 or type 2 diabetes. The two types are very different.

Type 1 diabetes

More than 15,000 children are diagnosed with type 1 diabetes each year in the United States. As noted in Chapter 1, in type 1 diabetes the pancreas produces little if any insulin. Without this hormone available to move blood sugar (glucose) into the body's muscles and tissues, excess glucose accumulates in the bloodstream. Left untreated, diabetes can cause serious organ damage and even death.

Signs and symptoms

Signs and symptoms of type 1 diabetes usually develop quickly — over a period of weeks — in children and teenagers. The first indication in babies and young children may be a yeast infection that causes a severe diaper rash. Fatigue or irritability is common and should raise your suspicion when associated with the most common warning signs and symptoms:

- Frequent urination
- Intense thirst
- Constant hunger
- Unexplained weight loss

Testing

If type 1 diabetes is suspected, your child's doctor will probably obtain a random blood glucose test at the

Wearing ID

No matter what the age, your child needs to wear an identification (ID) tag about diabetes so that others have access to emergency information when needed. Your teen may be more accepting if the ID is a necklace, dog tag or bracelet (for the wrist or ankle) that's unique and attractive. Even shoe tags for toddlers are available. You can search the Web for a variety of styles and prices, and many pharmacies also carry them. A wallet card can easily be overlooked and isn't carried all the time, so it may not help during sports activities, for example.

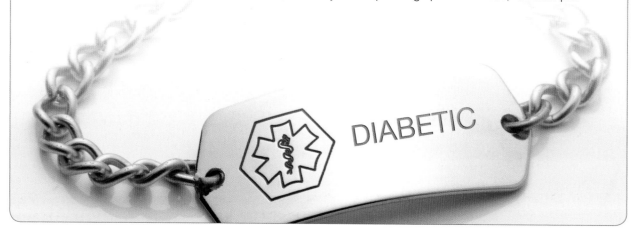

initial visit to check for an abnormally high level of glucose. Random means anytime of day, without the need for fasting. A result of 200 milligrams per deciliter (mg/dL) or greater will confirm the diagnosis.

In some circumstances, a doctor may recommend a fasting blood glucose test. Before having blood drawn for this test, your child will be instructed not to eat or drink for at least eight hours — typically, overnight.

After a fast, a blood glucose level under 100 mg/dL is considered normal. A glucose level from 100 to 125 mg/dL is called prediabetes, which indicates a high risk of developing diabetes. If it's 126 mg/dL or higher on two separate tests, a diagnosis of diabetes is likely.

If your child is diagnosed with type 1 diabetes, it's best to have an evaluation by an experienced diabetes team, including a pediatric endocrinologist — a doctor who specializes in treating children who have diabetes.

The doctor may order additional tests to check for a high ketone level in your child's urine or blood. Ketones are toxic acids that the body produces when it's not getting enough glucose and resorts to breaking down stored fat. Excess ketones can cause a life-threatening condition called diabetic ketoacidosis (kee-toe-ass-ih-DOE-sis), or DKA.

With prompt treatment this condition can be reversed. Children with DKA initially need treatment in a hospital. However, some children with mild DKA may be quickly and effectively treated with insulin therapy without the need for hospitalization.

Treatment

All people with type 1 diabetes, adults and children alike, depend on insulin therapy to live. Your child may take insulin with a syringe, an insulin pen or an insulin pump (see page 154).

The goal of insulin therapy is to bring blood glucose levels as near to normal as possible. Target blood glucose ranges for children and adolescents taking insulin may differ from the ranges set for adults.

Tight blood glucose control increases the risk of low blood glucose (hypoglycemia), and frequent instances of hypoglycemia can harm a young child's developing brain.

Near-normal blood glucose levels may be hard to achieve in children and teens. Your doctor will choose a blood glucose target range according to your child's medical needs and individual situation.

Before deciding to use an insulin pump, check your insurance provider for coverage. Pumps are more expensive than are injections, but many plans cover much of the cost.

The initial insulin dosage is based on weight, age, activity level and whether puberty has started. With the help of your doctor and diabetes educator, you and your child will learn how to make adjustments in insulin doses to manage expected changes in insulin needs as your child grows.

In children and teens, there are a few insulin regimens that are most often used.

Multiple daily injections (MDIs)

This regimen consists of a rapid- or short-acting insulin taken before meals and snacks as well as a long-acting insulin taken once a day to provide a baseline amount throughout the day.

Split-mixed program

This is a mixture of rapid- or short-acting insulin and intermediate-acting insulin in one injection, usually given twice each day.

Insulin pump

A programmable pump worn outside the body provides a continuous infusion of rapid- or short-acting insulin.

Studies show that insulin pumps are as safe and effective as injections are, even for many infants and toddlers. Ask your child's doctor how well the pump has worked for other children the same age as your son or daughter.

Type 2 diabetes

Type 2 diabetes used to be considered an adult disease. It was even referred to as adult-onset diabetes. Not anymore. Today, a significant number of type 2 cases are diagnosed in children. Why? Obesity plays a major role.

Over the past three decades, the rate of childhood obesity has more than doubled for children and teenagers. Those extra pounds carry an increased risk of type 2 diabetes. Today, most children and teenagers diagnosed with type 2 diabetes are overweight. Additional risk factors include:

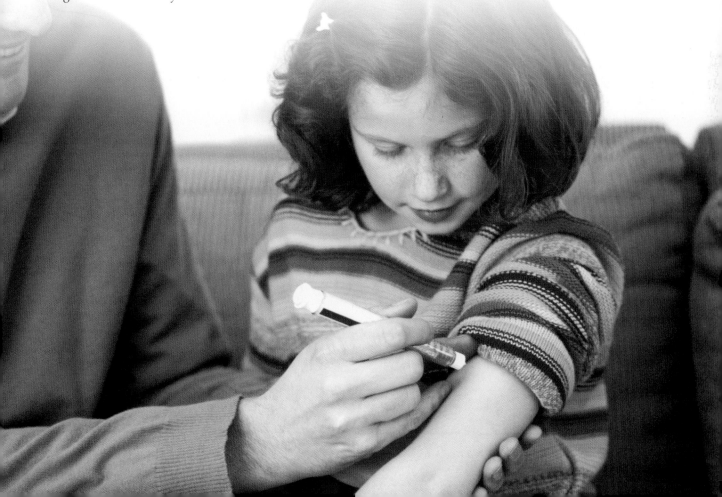

Puberty and diabetes

Just when you think you have a pretty good handle on helping your child control blood glucose, along comes puberty. Suddenly you're dealing with unpredictable moods and unpredictable blood glucose readings.

Some teenagers may start neglecting diabetes care as part of an overall drive for independence. This can play a role in unexplained high and low blood glucose readings during puberty. In addition, growth- and sex-hormone surges typically cause increased insulin resistance. Your teenager will probably need more insulin during puberty, along with more-frequent blood glucose tests to make sure that a mood swing isn't caused by hypoglycemia.

If your teenage daughter has higher blood glucose levels around the time of her period, you and your daughter should talk with her doctor. The doctor may adjust your daughter's treatment regimen to compensate for the influence of the menstrual cycle.

Your teen's self-sufficiency may tempt you to turn diabetes care entirely over to him or her. Don't do it. While it's important for your child to gradually assume more responsibility for diabetes management, parental guidance and support remains crucial to good diabetes control throughout the teen years. But remember that teenagers need to be fully prepared for taking over their diabetes care by the end of high school so that they're ready to handle it at college or wherever life takes them.

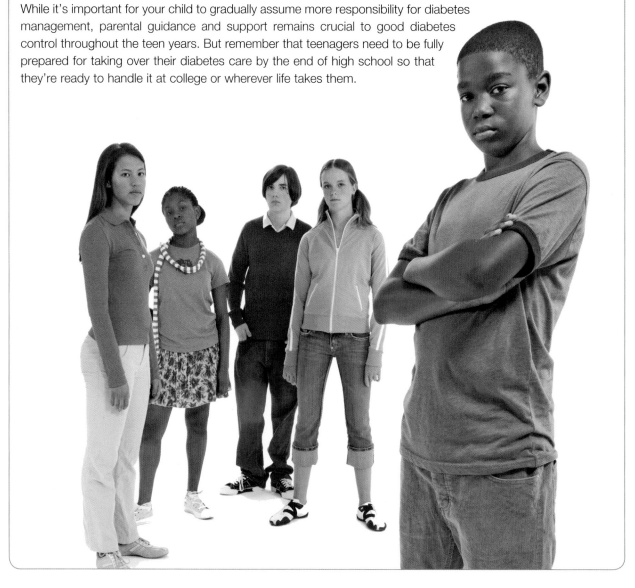

- **Family history.** Risk increases if a parent or sibling or other close relative has type 2 diabetes, but it's difficult to tell if this is learned behavior or genetics or both.
- **Race.** African-Americans, Hispanic-Americans, Native Americans, Asian-Americans and Pacific Islanders are at higher risk of diabetes for unclear reasons.
- **Signs of insulin resistance.** These are signs such as high blood pressure, polycystic ovarian syndrome or abnormal levels of blood fats (lipids).

Signs and symptoms

Unlike type 1 diabetes, in which symptoms typically develop quickly, the signs and symptoms of type 2 diabetes often appear gradually. These may include:

- Frequent urination
- Fatigue
- Intense thirst
- Blurred vision
- Constant hunger
- Frequent infections
- Unexplained weight loss
- Slow-healing sores

Some children with type 2 diabetes have patches of dark, velvety skin in the folds and creases of their bodies, usually in the armpits and neck. This condition, called acanthosis nigricans, is a sign of insulin resistance and increases the probability that your child has type 2 diabetes. However, many children with type 2 diabetes don't have any symptoms.

To diagnose the disease before it does serious damage, experts recommend testing all children and adolescents who are at high risk, even if they're symptom-free. One key risk factor is having a body mass index (BMI) greater than the 85th percentile for your child's age and sex. The BMI is a measurement based on a formula that takes into account weight and height to determine if your child has an unhealthy percentage of body fat.

Screening

If your child is overweight and has two of the risk factors previously noted — family history, high-risk race or signs of insulin resistance — ask your doctor about scheduling a diabetes screening.

Doctors usually use a fasting blood glucose test to diagnose type 2 diabetes in children. Your child will need to avoid food and liquid for at least eight hours before having blood drawn. If the test measures a blood glucose level of 126 mg/dL or higher on two separate tests, your child has diabetes.

Prediabetes

If a fasting blood glucose test indicates a level from 100 to 125 mg/dL, your child may be diagnosed with prediabetes. Many people with prediabetes eventually develop type 2 diabetes.

Studies show that adults with prediabetes who make dramatic improvements to their lifestyle, including eating healthier foods and exercising more, may prevent type 2 diabetes from developing. Children and teens with prediabetes can reduce their risk by making these same changes.

Ask your child's doctor for guidance. In addition, ask how often your child should be screened for diabetes. Whether your child has prediabetes or diabetes, developing healthy eating habits, increasing physical activity and getting regular exercise are vital to prevention and disease management.

Treatment

Some children and teenagers with type 2 diabetes can manage their blood glucose with diet and exercise along with oral drugs to lower blood glucose. In the United States, many children with type 2 diabetes also need insulin therapy. The decision about which treatment is best depends on the child, the level of blood glucose and whether the child has other health problems.

Metformin is the only oral medication that's approved for children and adolescents (age 10 and older) with type 2 diabetes. It's an effective option for many people with diabetes, but some brands are only for use in adults. In addition, metformin isn't safe for anyone with liver, kidney or heart failure, and it may cause gastrointestinal problems. For more information on metformin see page 157.

Caring for medical needs

Leaving your child in the care of someone else can be nerve-wracking for any parent. If your child has diabetes, you might be even more fearful. But both you and your child are likely to feel more secure knowing that people outside the family can be relied on to help manage diabetes with your child. And your child will build self-confidence from handling diabetes care when you're not around. So take a deep breath, and then take action.

Creating a diabetes care plan

Sit down with your diabetes educator to create a care plan that maps out your child's treatment regimen and how to respond to high or low blood glucose. Then, meet with school or child care personnel to go over the plan in detail.

Note the names of adults who will be primarily responsible for helping your child check his or her blood glucose and take medications. This usually involves a talk with the school nurse. Ask the school nurse or an administrator to help you share the plan with all adults who'll be supervising your child during the day, including teachers, office staff, coaches and bus drivers.

Your child's diabetes educator or doctor may be able to help you train school and child care staff to perform diabetes care tasks, if they already aren't able to do so.

Blood glucose monitoring

Regular blood glucose tests are the only way to know with confidence whether your child's treatment program is working. Whether they have type 1 or type 2 diabetes, children and teenagers who use insulin may need four or more blood glucose checks each day. Your child's doctor can help you determine the best testing schedule.

Each time you perform a blood glucose test, log the results in a record book. Keep a separate record book at your child's school for tracking results during the day. Young children will need an adult's help to maintain school record books, but children age 8 and older may be able to log results on their own.

The information you record will help you see how food, physical activity, illness and other factors affect your child's blood glucose. You may start to see patterns that will help your doctor develop the best treatment program for your child.

Young children in particular may have a hard time recognizing the signs and symptoms of low blood glucose (hypoglycemia), explained in Chapter 2. Teach your child — and any caregivers — that if there's any doubt, check the blood glucose.

Regardless of his or her age, getting used to frequent glucose checks can be challenging for your child — and for you. Focus on reassuring (rather than scolding) your child when he or she resists testing because it's uncomfortable. Allow your young child to make some decisions, even if it's as simple as choosing the spot for the glucose check.

Consider simple rewards, such as stickers (not food). Ask your health care team how to approach this task, including how to deal with the emotional challenges you may face.

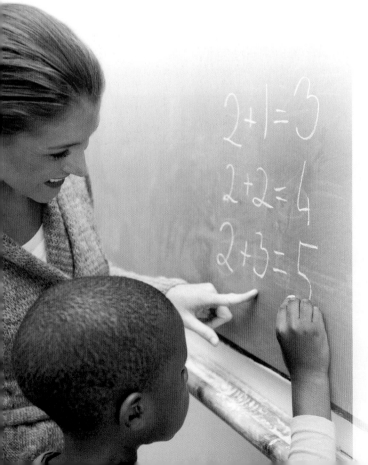

Involving your child

Encourage your child's active participation in meetings and discussions about diabetes care. Eventually, your child will need to take on total responsibility for managing diabetes. You can start working toward that goal from the beginning by asking your child to help with care tasks in age-appropriate ways.

The extent to which your child is ready to participate depends on age, abilities and willingness. Here's a general idea of what you can aim for, but ask your child's doctor for guidance because children develop at different rates.

Ages 2 through 3

Your child may be able to pick out a test strip for a blood glucose test, choose between two places for an injection or wipe off the injection site with a swab.

Ages 4 through 7

Your child may be able to help keep blood glucose records and may enjoy helping plan healthy meals and games or outings that encourage physical activity for the family.

Ages 8 through 11

With supervision and support, your child may be able to perform a finger-stick blood glucose test by age 8 and self-administer insulin by age 10.

Ages 12 through 15

This age group may be ready to self-monitor blood glucose levels under normal circumstances. A child who takes insulin should be able to manage injections or pump infusions with supervision.

Ages 16 through 18

Your daughter or son should be ready to start managing diabetes care independently as a teenager so that he or she can take over the responsibility by the end of high school. This includes being well-prepared to respond to possible blood sugar complications such as hypoglycemia or hyperglycemia.

Blood sugar vs. blood glucose

You'll likely hear the term *blood sugar* more often than *blood glucose*. The terms mean the same thing.

If you decide to use the term *blood sugar*, make sure that your child understands what it means (explained in Chapter 1). Eating other types of carbohydrates — not just sugary foods — can make blood sugar (glucose) rise. Even some adults who've had diabetes for many years still think they can't eat any sugar. But they don't realize they're eating too much of other foods that can make their blood glucose rise. The key is moderation.

For the full story on healthy eating, see Chapter 3, including The scoop on sugar, page 64.

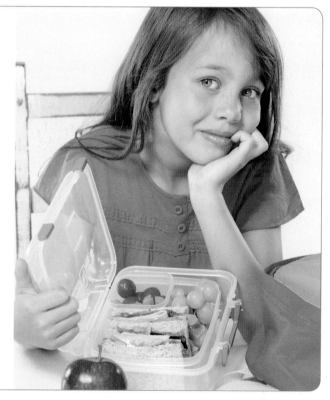

Emotional and social issues

Coping with a diagnosis of diabetes is tough for all children and teens. If your child is very young, all the tests and injections may feel like punishment. An older child may be crushed to realize that he or she is different from peers and that diabetes isn't going to go away.

Sadness, anger and withdrawal are all normal reactions. However, feelings of hopelessness that last for weeks call for medical attention.

Encourage your child to talk about feelings. Your preschooler may be able to vent emotions by drawing pictures or role-playing with dolls and stuffed animals. Older children may feel better just having a chance to holler, stomp, kick a pillow or cry. (Parents, too!)

Listen to your child without trying to put a positive spin on diabetes. Let your son or daughter know that you're there to help. Your child may be nervous about telling friends about the diagnosis. Volunteer for practice conversations, and let your child know that whom to tell, when to tell and how much to say is up to him or her — it's a personal decision.

Your child may want to talk with a trusted teacher or school social worker who can help ease the transition to managing diabetes at school. A local support group, online forum or camp (see page 217) for children and teens with diabetes also might make coping easier. Your diabetes educator can put you in touch with resources.

When it's more than sadness

Diabetes increases the risk of depression. Watch for these signs and symptoms in your son or daughter:

▶ Not caring about the things he or she used to
▶ Having trouble sleeping
▶ Staying in bed all the time
▶ Eating a lot more or eating less than usual
▶ Losing or gaining a lot of weight without trying
▶ Difficulty concentrating
▶ Having anxiety
▶ Crying a lot
▶ Expressing a desire to hurt oneself or to die

If you think your child may be depressed, seek help right away. Your doctor or diabetes educator can refer your child to a mental health professional.

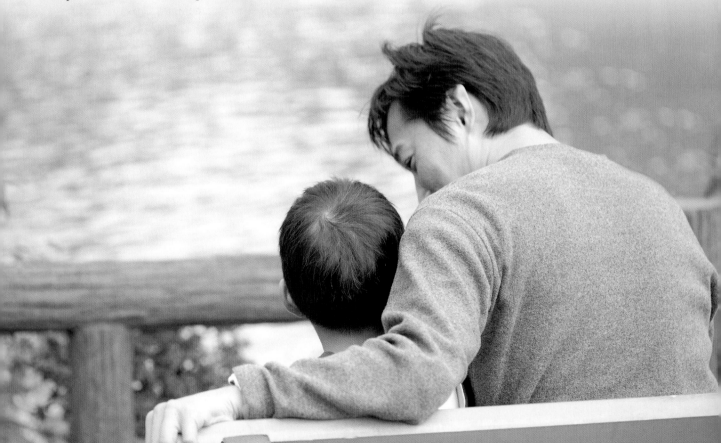

Diabetes and drinking: A dangerous mix

Your teenager is headed out to a party with friends. Like most parents, you worry about whether alcohol will be served and whether your child will make smart choices if friends are drinking. Have a frank discussion with your teenager about the risks of alcohol. Alcohol increases the risk of hypoglycemia, and the sugar content of many mixed drinks can raise blood glucose. If your teenager experiences high or low blood glucose while partying with friends, they may think your child is drunk and take no action to help. It's just not worth the risk. Talk to your child about ways to say no if pressured to drink.

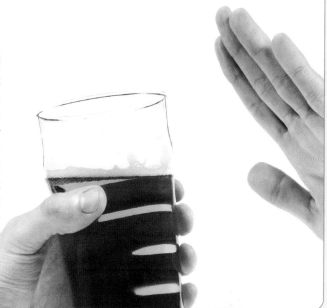

? Are teenage girls with diabetes at higher risk of eating disorders?

Yes. According to the American Diabetes Association, teenage girls with type 1 diabetes may be twice as likely as their peers who don't have diabetes to develop eating disorders. This includes gradually starving themselves (anorexia) and forcing themselves to throw up after eating (bulimia).

It may be that having to pay such close attention to food makes girls with diabetes more likely to obsess about their weight. And insulin can be manipulated to cause weight loss. Eating disorders increase the risk of complications from diabetes. Even in teens without diabetes, eating disorders can be fatal.

Signs that your daughter may have an eating disorder include:

▶ Extreme fluctuations in blood glucose that can't be explained
▶ Frequent problems with high or low blood glucose
▶ Not complying with insulin needs
▶ Obsession with food or with losing weight
▶ Avoiding being weighed
▶ Wearing baggy clothes to hide weight loss
▶ Avoiding meals with the family
▶ Binge eating
▶ Excessive exercising
▶ Irregular menstrual periods or no menstrual periods

If you think your daughter may have an eating disorder, call her doctor. The doctor may arrange for your daughter to see a mental health professional with special training in eating disorders.

Good habits for staying healthy

Healthy eating, increased physical activity and regularly monitoring your blood sugar are key steps to managing diabetes.

Your positive attitude and active participation is a crucial part of helping your child make these permanent lifestyle changes.

Tips for healthy eating

It's recommended that people with diabetes follow the same healthy-eating plan recommended for everyone, with moderate portions at regular mealtimes.

That means eating a variety of fresh fruits and vegetables, whole grains, and fat-free or low-fat dairy products. It also means fewer fried foods, burgers, sodas, prepackaged muffins and other unhealthy foods. See Chapter 3 for more information.

Chances are, your entire family would benefit from making the same improvements to fuel up for a healthy, active life.

Launch a family project to find tempting, low-fat recipes. Schedule a movie night and set nutritious snacks on the coffee table. Try air-popped popcorn, fat-free or low-fat chips with salsa, veggies with hummus dip, seasoned and baked potato skins, and fruit-and-yogurt parfaits.

Here are some tips for enlisting the whole family in a healthy-eating program:

◗ Involve your children in helping to prepare meals in age-appropriate ways. They're much more likely to try a new vegetable dish if they helped chop up the ingredients.

◗ Eat as many family meals together as possible, and keep table conversation to pleasant topics.

◗ Don't deprive your child or your family of enjoying a dessert, but choose healthier foods. Modify a favorite recipe with the help of your dietitian, try new recipes, and always use appropriate portions. A carefully chosen dessert at the end of a balanced meal is fine every once in a while, and it can help reduce the likelihood that your child will feel deprived.

◗ Work with your dietitian to include allowances for foods that your family usually enjoys at special celebrations or occasions.

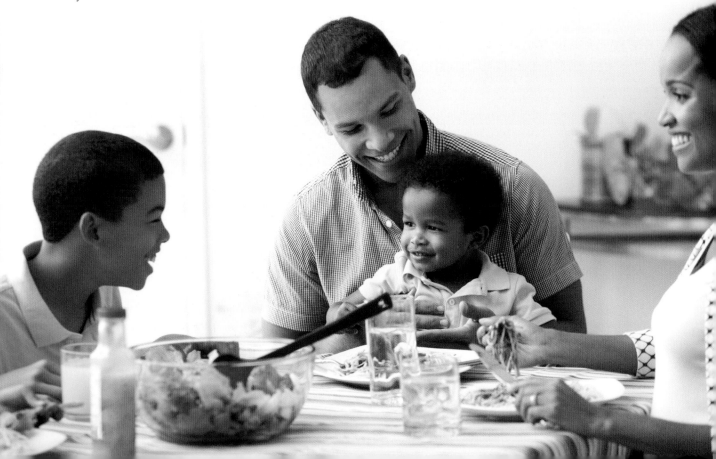

No limits to achievement

If you worry that diabetes might limit the dreams your child can reach for, consider Gary Hall Jr.'s story. Gary had four Olympic swimming medals in his pocket and was training for more when, in 1999, he started noticing that he was always thirsty and his vision was blurred. He was soon diagnosed with type 1 diabetes. Gary was shocked. There was no history of diabetes in his family, and he had always worked hard to keep in excellent physical condition.

Gary decided he wasn't going to let diabetes stop him. He found a doctor who believed it was possible for him to continue to train and compete. Under his doctor's supervision, Gary dedicated himself to a rigorous schedule of blood glucose testing and treatment and got back in the pool. At the 2000 Olympic games in Sydney, Australia, Gary won four more medals. And at the 2004 games in Athens, Greece, he took gold in the 50-meter freestyle and became one of the most decorated Olympic athletes in history.

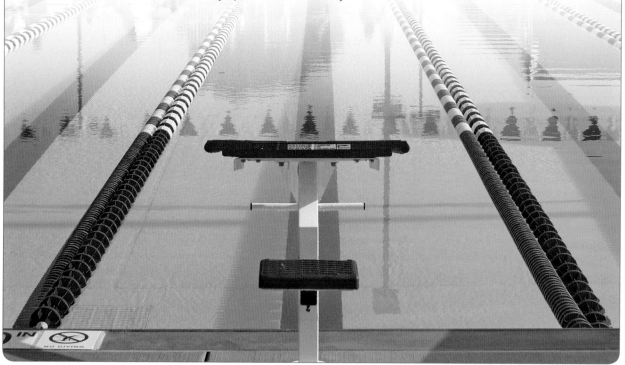

Eating away from home

Find out if healthy foods are on the menu in your child's school cafeteria. If they're not, pack a lunch that follows the same nutritious standards you're setting for the family dinner table. Then call the school and encourage better options.

Most children and teenagers also need a couple of snacks during the day. Ward off vending machine temptations by slipping tasty, wholesome options into your child's backpack. Smart snack choices include:

- Fat-free or low-fat crackers with low-fat cheese
- Whole-grain bread with peanut butter
- A small tortilla lightly topped with low-fat cheese or turkey
- Fresh fruit

If your child is planning a sleepover at a friend's house, call the other parents and — with your child's permission — discuss what food will be served and why you're asking. If they're not planning healthy snacks, tell them you'll send some with your child, and include enough for the other children to enjoy.

Getting more physically active

Getting active with your child is an essential part of making exercise habits stick, and it will improve your health, too. While regular exercise is important, any physical activity has health benefits. Here are just a few easy ideas to get your whole family moving:

▶ Head out for a walk and explore the sights together.
▶ Whip the yard into shape — rake leaves, garden or shovel snow.
▶ Throw a ball or a Frisbee disc around.
▶ Go bicycling or in-line skating.
▶ Turn up the radio or stereo and have an impromptu dance party.
▶ If you have young children, get out the chalk and play hopscotch or duck down for a game of hide-and-seek.

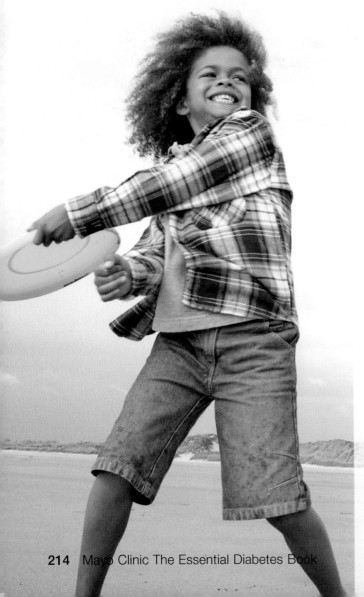

Blood sugar monitoring

Depending on your child's treatment plan, you may need to check and record your child's blood sugar several times a day. This requires frequent finger sticks. But it's the only way to make sure that your child's blood sugar level remains within his or her target range — which may change as your child grows and changes.

Even if your child eats on a rigid schedule, the amount of sugar in his or her blood can change unpredictably. With help from your child's diabetes treatment team, you'll learn how your child's blood sugar level changes in response to:

▶ **Food.** What and how much your child eats will affect your child's blood sugar level. Blood sugar is typically highest one to two hours after a meal.
▶ **Physical activity.** Physical activity moves sugar from your child's blood into his or her cells. The more active your child is, the lower his or her blood sugar level.
▶ **Medication.** Any medications your child takes may affect his or her blood sugar level, sometimes requiring changes in your child's diabetes treatment plan.
▶ **Illness.** During a cold or other illness, your child's body will produce hormones that raise his or her blood sugar level.

Additional test

In addition to frequent blood sugar monitoring, your child's doctor may recommend regular A1C testing. An A1C test, also known as a glycated hemoglobin test, is a blood test that indicates your child's average blood sugar level for the past two to three months.

It works by measuring the percentage of blood sugar attached to hemoglobin, the oxygen-carrying protein in red blood cells. The higher your child's blood sugar levels, the more hemoglobin he or she will have with sugar attached. Your child's target A1C goal may vary depending on his or her age and various other factors.

Compared with repeated daily blood sugar tests, A1C testing better indicates how well your child's diabetes treatment plan is working. An elevated A1C level may signal the need for a change in your child's treatment plan.

Surviving sick days

Every child has a day here and there when he or she is sick — kids with diabetes are no exception. How do you care for your child during illness? Follow these tips from the American Diabetes Association.

Continue insulin treatment

Your intuition might tell you to reduce or stop your child's insulin, especially if he or she isn't eating much. Younger or newly diagnosed children could need reduced insulin depending on their blood glucose levels, but other children need just the opposite — extra insulin. Ask your doctor for guidelines for insulin treatment on sick days, and call the doctor if you're not sure how much insulin to give.

Stay close to the meal plan

You may want to substitute soup and other comfort foods for the usual fare. Just be sure to maintain about the same mealtimes and ratio of carbohydrates at each meal and snack as you would on a normal day.

If your child has an upset stomach and can't eat, give him or her clear liquids that contain carbohydrates (sports drinks, juices, gelatin, frozen fruit bars).

Give plenty of liquids

Encourage your child to drink water and other non-caffeinated beverages.

Choose medications wisely

Many over-the-counter medications contain sugar, alcohol or both. Although there might not be too much sugar in one dose of cough syrup, it can add up if your child takes the medicine every four hours. If you can't find a sugar-free version or if it's more expensive, just account for the medicine's carbohydrates in the meal plan.

Medicines that contain alcohol can lower blood glucose levels. If you give your child a medicine that contains alcohol, have him or her eat something while taking it in order to prevent hypoglycemia. Or you may want to find an option that is alcohol-free.

In addition, certain medications can affect your child's diabetes. Many decongestants, for example, can raise blood glucose levels. Ask the doctor what over-the-counter medications he or she recommends for common ailments.

Check blood glucose and ketone levels frequently

Diabetic ketoacidosis (DKA) is a danger whenever your child is sick. DKA occurs when a person with diabetes has too little insulin in his or her system. If left untreated, DKA can lead to coma.

To prevent DKA or catch it early, check your child's blood glucose levels often (every few hours). Also, check your child's urine for ketones several times a day. If he or she is vomiting or has diarrhea, check ketones even more frequently.

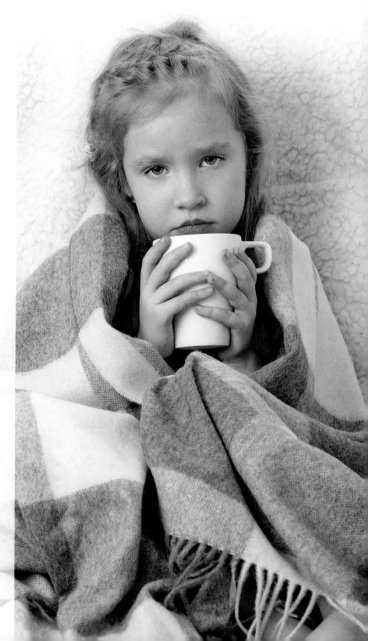

Foods for sick days

When your child isn't feeling well, he or she may not feel like eating much. But it's important for your child to eat in order to keep his or her body from burning fats for fuel (and making ketones) and to keep the body energized so that it can get better fast.

Here are a few flu-friendly food ideas for when a bug has your child down. These foods contain between 10 and 15 grams of carbohydrates.

Fluids
- 1 double-stick Popsicle
- 1 cup Gatorade
- 1 cup milk
- 1 cup soup
- ½ cup fruit juice
- ½ cup regular soft drink (not diet)

Foods
- 6 saltines
- 5 vanilla wafers
- 4 Lifesavers
- 3 graham crackers
- 1 slice dry toast (not light bread)
- ½ cup cooked cereal
- ⅓ cup frozen yogurt
- ½ cup regular ice cream
- ½ cup sugar-free pudding
- ½ cup regular (not sugar-free) gelatin dessert
- ½ cup custard
- ½ cup mashed potatoes
- ¼ cup sherbet
- ¼ cup regular pudding

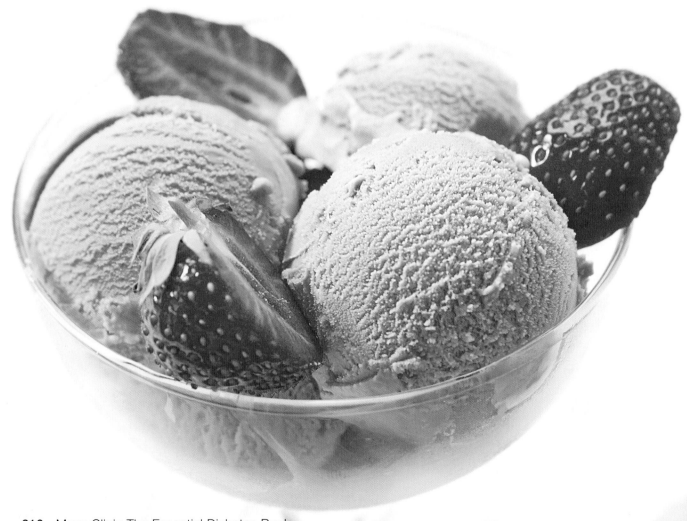

Diabetes camps

Think your child would savor the chance to hang out with other kids who have diabetes? Look into a diabetes camp provided by the American Diabetes Association. Staff members are trained in diabetes care, and part of their time with campers is focused on sharing tips for good diabetes management. But a lot of time at camp is spent just having fun with friends who'll make your child feel ordinary — in the best possible way. Ask your diabetes educator to help you locate camps near you.

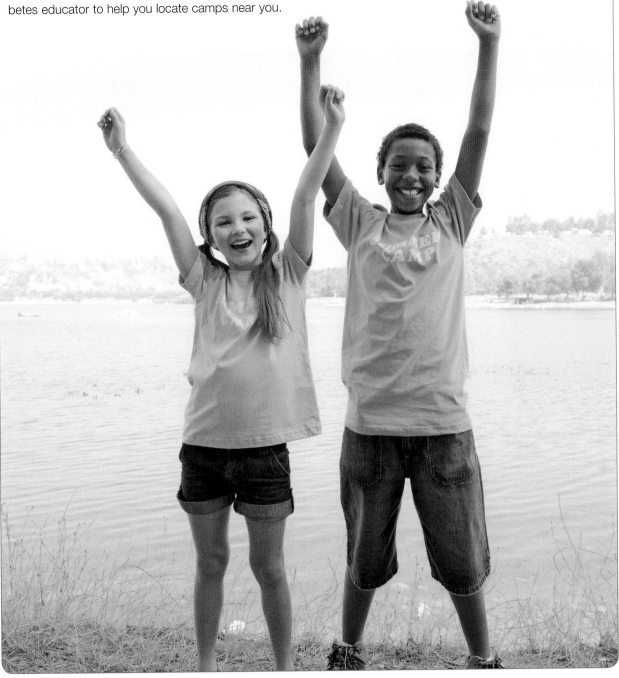

Additional Resources

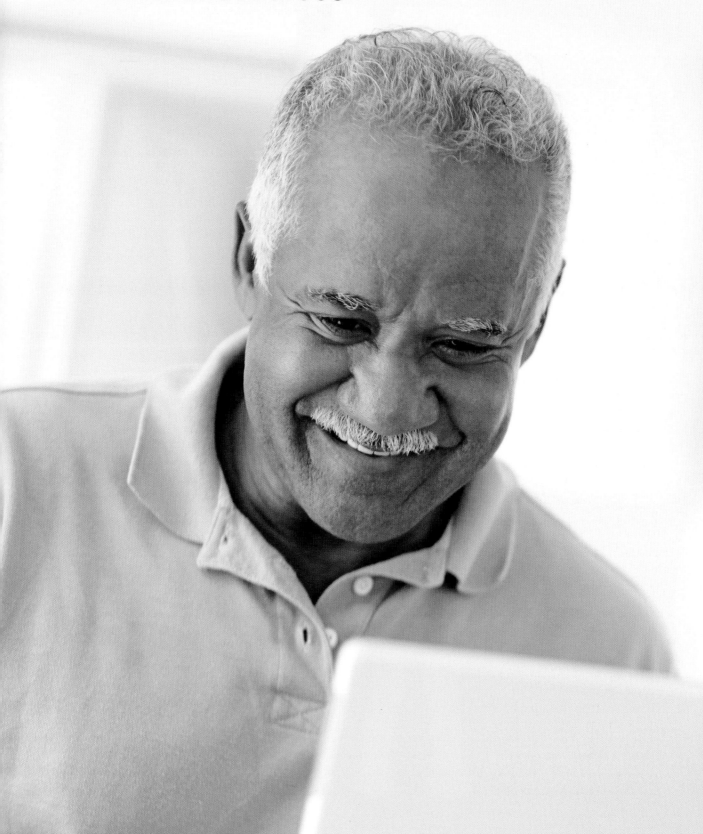

American Association of Acupuncture and Oriental Medicine
P.O. Box 96503 No. 44114
Washington, DC 20090-6503
866-455-7999
www.aaaomonline.org

American Association of Diabetes Educators
200 W. Madison St.
Suite 800
Chicago, IL 60606
800-338-3633
www.diabeteseducator.org

American Diabetes Association
1701 N. Beauregard St.
Alexandria, VA 22311
800-DIABETES (800-342-2383)
www.diabetes.org

Canadian Diabetes Association
1400-522 University Ave.
Toronto, ON M5G 2R5
Canada
800-226-8464
www.diabetes.ca

Centers for Disease Control and Prevention, Division of Diabetes Translation
1600 Clifton Road
Atlanta, GA 30333
800-232-4636
www.cdc.gov/diabetes

Insulindependence
249 S. Hwy 101
Suite 8000
Solana Beach, CA 92075
888-912-3837
www.insulindependence.org

International Diabetes Federation
166 Chaussee de La Hulpe
B-1170 Brussels
Belgium
32-2-5385511
www.idf.org

JDRF (formerly Juvenile Diabetes Research Foundation International)
26 Broadway
New York, NY 10004
800-533-CURE (800-533-2873)
www.jdrf.org

Mayo Clinic
www.MayoClinic.org
Search for *diabetes* and related terms

National Diabetes Education Program
1 Diabetes Way
Bethesda, MD 20814-9692
301-496-3583
www.ndep.nih.gov

National Diabetes Information Clearinghouse
1 Information Way
Bethesda, MD 20892-3560
800-860-8747
www.diabetes.niddk.nih.gov

National Kidney Disease Education Program
3 Kidney Information Way
Bethesda, MD 20892
866-4-KIDNEY (866-454-3639)
www.nkdep.nih.gov

National Kidney Foundation
30 E. 33rd St.
New York, NY 10016
800-622-9010
www.kidney.org

Scientific Registry of Transplant Recipients
914 S. 8th St.
Suite S-4.100
Minneapolis, MN 55404
877-970-7787
www.srtr.org

United Network for Organ Sharing
P.O. Box 2484
Richmond, VA 23218
888-894-6361
www.unos.org

Index

A

abdomen, insulin injections in, 149
activities
  aerobic, 113
  as eating triggers, 103
  leisure, 188–189
activity logs, 134
aerobic exercise
  activities, 113
  defined, 122
  examples of, 122
  intensity, gauging, 123
  starting, 122
  walking, 124–127
age, as risk factor, 18
alcohol
  blood glucose levels and, 44
  childhood diabetes and, 211
  diabetes and, 66
alpha-glucosidase inhibitors, 158–159, 160
alprostadil, 198
alternate site testing, 36, 37
A1C test
  childhood diabetes and, 214
  defined, 20, 174
  frequency of, 174–175
  functioning of, 174
  how it helps, 175

B

barriers
  blood glucose monitoring, 49
  exercise, 120–121
  weight loss, 90–91
beverages, calories of, 102
biguanides, 157, 158–159
birth defects, 190
blood glucose
  blood sugar vs., 209
  processing of, 10–11
  sources of, 10
  too much, 10
blood glucose levels
  alcohol and, 45
  carbohydrates and, 54
  exercise/physical activity and, 44
  factors affecting, 43–46
  food and, 43
  illness and, 44
  keeping within range, 40
  liver and, 43
  medications and, 44
  plasma glucose levels vs., 37
  stress and, 46
blood glucose meters
  calibration, 41
  checking, 41
  choosing, 34
  defined, 33
  troubleshooting, 41
blood glucose monitoring
  advanced tools for, 36–37
  alternate site testing, 36, 37
  approach to, 31–32
  barriers, overcoming, 49
  childhood diabetes, 208

continuous glucose monitor, 36
cost and, 49
disposable glucose monitor, 36
exercise and, 136–137
fear and, 49
goals, 40
health care access and, 49
lancet and lancing device, 33
lifestyle issues, 49
meters, 33, 34
numbers game and, 40
performing, 35
pregnancy and, 190–191
privacy issues, 49
problems, troubleshooting, 41–42
within range, 40
recommendations from experts, 35
results signaling a problem, 46
technique, checking, 42
testing basics, 35
testing frequency, 32–33
test strips, 33
tracking results, 38
type 1 childhood diabetes, 204
blood pressure
  checking, 173
  goals and treatment, 178
  monitoring, 178
blood sugar
  blood glucose vs., 209
  control, 148
  monitoring, childhood diabetes and, 214
blurred vision, 16
body mass index (BMI), 86–87, 88
breathing, relaxed, 185

C

calories
  in beverages, 102
  burned per hour, 127
  controlling, 61
  daily serving recommendations for, 97
  goal, determining, 96
carbohydrates
  counting, 62–63
  on food labels, 61
  function of, 53
  glucose level and, 54
  myths and facts, 54
  sweets and, 64
cardiovascular disease, 26–27
checkups
  blood and urine tests, 174
  blood pressure, 173
  expectations at, 173–174
  feet, 173–174
  weight, 173
childhood diabetes
  achievement and, 213
  blood glucose monitoring, 208
  blood sugar monitoring, 214
  care plan, 208
  child involvement and, 209
  depression and, 210
  diabetes camps, 217
  drinking and, 211
  eating disorders and, 211
  emotional and social issues, 200–201
  habits for staying healthy, 212–214
  medical needs, caring for, 208–209

sick days, 215–216
statistics, 201
type 1, 203–205
type 2, 205–207
cholesterol, 175, 178
complications, long term
  eye damage (retinopathy), 28–29
  heart and blood disease, 26–27
  kidney disease (nephropathy), 28
  nerve damage (neuropathy), 27–28
  stroke, 27
continuous glucose monitor, 36
continuous subcutaneous insulin infusion
  (CSII), 155
cookbooks, 106
cooling down, 135
coronary artery disease, 26
counting carbs, 62
CSII. See continuous subcutaneous
  insulin infusion)

D

daily food record, 97
daily serving recommendations, 97
dehydration, avoiding, 128
depression, childhood diabetes and, 211
diabetes
  alcohol and, 66
  carb counting and, 62–63
  childhood, 200–217
  dangers, 21
  defined, 10–11
  gestational, 13, 192–193
  heart attacks and, 21
  LADA, 15
  long-term complications, 26–29
  metabolic syndrome and, 19
  MODY, 15
  as national epidemic, 11
  physical activity and, 113
  puberty and, 206
  signs and symptoms, 15–16
  statistics, 9, 11
  tests for detection, 20–21
  warning signs, 15
  See also type 1 diabetes; type 2 diabetes
diabetes camps, 217
diabetes diet, 52
diabetes identification, wearing, 153
diabetes insipidus, 11
diabetes mellitus, 11
diabetic coma, 23
diabetic ketoacidosis (DKA), 23–24, 25
diabetic retinopathy, 28–29
diet. See healthy eating
dietitians, 57
disposable glucose monitor, 36
DKA. See diabetic ketoacidosis
DPP-4 inhibitors, 158–159, 161
  metformin and, 162
  See also oral medications

E

eating disorders, childhood diabetes and, 211
eating triggers, 103
energy density
  fiber, 98
  high, 98–99
  low, 98–99
  water, 98

erectile dysfunction and diabetes, 196–199
exams
eye, 179
list of, 177
exchange lists in, 65
exenatide (Byetta, Bydureon), 164
exercise(s)
activity log, 134
aerobic, 122–124
amount of, 129
barriers, tackling, 120–121
best time for, 139
blood glucose levels and, 44
building up gradually, 129
calories burned per hour, 127
clothing and shoes, 135
defined, 114
environment, 135
feet and, 135
fluids and, 135
hydration and, 128
injury avoidance, 135
intensity, gauging, 123
motivation, 137–139
physical activity vs., 114
plateaus, 139
positive self-talk and, 138
progress, monitoring, 137
regular monitoring and, 136–137
strengthening, 132–134
stretching, 130–131
warming up/cooling down, 135
warning signs of when to stop, 129
weight training, 133
See also fitness; physical activity
external eye exam, 179
eye damage (retinopathy), 28–29
eye doctors (ophthalmologists or
optometrists), 172
eyes, caring for, 179

F
family history, as risk factor, 17
fasting blood glucose test, 20–21
fats
good and bad, 55
reducing amount of, 106
saturated, 55, 56
tips for limiting, 55
feet
blood flow, 180
caring for, 180–182
checking, 173–174, 180
exercise and, 135
products for, 181
shoes and, 181–182
socks and, 180
toenails, 181
fiber, 98
fitness
activities, choosing, 119
assessing, 116
breaks, 118
as essential to health and well-being,
115–116
keeping physically active and, 118
for kids, 140–141
motivation, 117
personal plan, creating, 117
score, 116

flu-like feeling, 15
flu shots, 184
food labels, 61
food record, 97, 101–102
food(s)
blood glucose levels and, 43
as eating triggers, 103
fresh, at store perimeter, 107
shopping for, 107
for sick days, 216
foot doctors (podiatrists), 172, 181

G
gestational diabetes, 13, 192–193
glimepiride (Amaryl), 156
glipizide (Glucotrol), 156
glucose, during digestion, 10
glyburide (DiaBeta, Glynase), 156
glycated hemoglobin test. See A1C test
glycemic index, 62
goals
blood pressure, 178
calorie, 96
children and teens with type 1 diabetes, 203
insulin therapy, 144
weight training, 133
goals, weight loss
reassessing and adjusting, 93
re-evaluating, 110
rewards, 93
setting, 92–93
SMART, 92–93
gum disease, 16

H
health
eye, 179
fitness and, 115
foot, 180–182
men's, 196–199
stress management, 185–189
teeth, 183
vaccinations, 184
women's, 190–196
yearly checkups and, 173–174
health care team, 172
healthy eating
for all types of diabetes, 53
calorie control and, 61
carb counting and, 62–63
carbohydrates and, 53–54, 61
childhood diabetes and, 212–213
consistency, 51
decisions, 68
defined, 52–53
diabetes diet and, 52
exchange lists in, 65
fats and, 54–56
food labels and, 61
meal planning, 57–59
motivation, 67
omega-3s and, 56
plate method, 60
protein and, 54
questions for, 51
recipes, 68–83
rewards, 67
serving sizes, 58–59
sugar-free products and, 61
sweets and, 64

healthy weight
achieving, 84–111
benefits of, 85
body mass index (BMI) and, 86–87
determination, 86–88
eating triggers and, 103
energy density and, 98–100
getting back on track, 109–110
habits for a lifetime, 110
Mayo Clinic Healthy Weight Pyramid, 95–97
meal routine and, 104–105
personal history and, 88
setbacks, overcoming, 109–111
simple first steps, 94
smart shopping and, 107
tools for goal evaluation, 111
type 2 diabetes and, 85–86
waist circumference and, 87
willpower vs. self-control and, 108
See also weight loss
heart attacks, 21, 26–27
hemodialysis, 165, 166
herbal remedies, 157
high blood sugar
avoiding, 46–47
defined, 23
handling, 25
prevention steps, 47
response to, 47
high ketones (diabetic ketoacidosis), 23–24, 25
hunger, shopping and, 107
hydration, 128, 135
hyperglycemia, 23, 25
hypoglycemia, 21–23, 25
as pregnancy complication, 194

I
identification (ID) tags, 204
illness, blood glucose levels and, 44
implantable insulin pumps, 156
inactivity, as risk factor, 17–18
infections, 16
injectable drugs, 164
injury avoidance, 135
insulin
changes in appearance, 153
drawing into syringe, 150
function of, 10
intermediate-acting, 146–147
long-acting, 146–147
metformin and, 163
options, 146–147
oral medications and, 162–163
pre-mixed, 144
problems, avoiding, 153
purchasing, 153
rapid-acting, 146–147
short-acting, 146–147
storing, 153
sulfonylureas and, 162–163
type 2 diabetes and, 163
types of, 144
TZD and, 163
insulin injections
in abdomen, 149
insulin in syringe, 150
process, 151
site problems, avoiding, 151
site selection, 149
syringe and needle alternatives, 152

insulin pumps
  benefits of, 155
  candidates for, 155
  correct use of, 156
  defined, 145, 154
  implantable, 156
  infusion site, changing, 154
  type 1 childhood diabetes, 205
insulin therapy
  complications, preventing, 148
  defined, 144
  goals, 144
  intensive, 145–148
  mixed dose, 145
  pre-mixed dose, 145
  regimens, 145
  single dose, 145
  split dose, 145
  split mixed dose, 145
  split pre-mixed dose, 145
  team approach, 148
intensive insulin therapy
  combination of insulins, 145
  complications, preventing, 148
  defined, 145
  drawbacks to, 148
  multiple daily injections, 145
  team approach, 148
intermediate-acting insulin, 146–147
islet cell transplant, 168–169

K
kidney dialysis, 165–166
kidney disease (nephropathy), 28
kidney transplant, 167, 168
kids, fitness for, 140–141

L
lancet and lancing device, 33
latent autoimmune diabetes of adults (LADA),
  15
lipid panel, 175–176
liquid meal replacements, 108
liraglutide (Victoza), 164
liver, blood glucose levels and, 43
long-acting insulin, 146–147
low blood glucose, insulin pumps and, 155
low blood sugar
  avoiding, 48–49
  handling, 25
  as medical emergency, 21–23
  prevention steps, 49
  response to, 48–49
  what to watch for, 48

M
massage, 187–188
maturity-onset diabetes of youth (MODY), 15
Mayo Clinic Healthy Weight Pyramid
  carbohydrates, 96
  defined, 95
  fats, 96
  food groups, 96
  fruits, 96
  illustrated, 95
  physical activity and, 95, 97
  protein and dairy, 96
  sweets, 96
  tailoring, 96–97
  vegetables, 96

meal planning
  consistency and, 58
  counting carbs and, 62–63
  with dietitian, 57
  exchange lists in, 65
  glycemic index and, 62
  overview of, 57
  variety and, 58
  See also healthy eating
meals
  liquid replacements, 108
  number per day, 104
  routines, 104–105
  See also healthy eating; healthy weight
medical emergencies
  handling, 25
  high blood sugar (hyperglycemia), 23
  ketones (diabetic ketoacidosis), 23–24
  low blood sugar (hypoglycemia), 21–23
medical history, in healthy weight
  determination, 88
medical treatment
  injectable drugs, 164
  insulin injections, 149–152
  with insulin pumps, 154–156
  insulin therapy, 145–148
  kidney dialysis, 165–166
  kidney transplant, 167
  oral diabetes medications, 156–161
  problems, avoiding, 153
  purpose of, 143
  transplant procedures, 167–169
medications. See injectable drugs; insulin;
  oral medications
meditation, 187
meglitinides, 158–159, 160–161
  See also oral medications
menopause and diabetes, 195–196
men's health, 196–199
menstruation, 195
metabolic syndrome, 19
metformin, 157, 158–159
  DPP-4 inhibitors and, 162
  insulin and, 163
  sulfonylurea and, 162
  TZDs and, 162
motivation
  exercise, 137–139
  healthy eating and, 67
  walking, 125

N
nephropathy, 28
nerve damage (neuropathy), 27–28
neuropathy, 27–28
nurses, 172
nutrition labels, reading, 107

O
omega-3s, 56
oral glucose tolerance test, 21
oral medications
  alpha-glucosidase inhibitors, 160
  biguanides, 156–157
  blood glucose levels and, 44
  checking, 153
  combination pills, 162
  combinations of, 162
  DPP-4 inhibitors, 161
  factors affecting, 156

insulin and, 162–163
  meglitinides, 160–161
  sulfonylureas, 156–157
  summary, 158–159
  TZDs, 160
  See also insulin; insulin injections

P
pancreas transplant, 167–168
pedometers, 114
peritoneal dialysis, 165–166
physical activity
  blood glucose levels and, 44
  calories burned per hour, 127
  childhood diabetes and, 214
  choosing, 119
  in diabetes management, 113
  doctor consultation before starting, 113
  every move counts, 114
  exercise vs., 114
  fitting into home life, 118
  recommendation, 129
  Mayo Clinic Healthy Weight Pyramid and,
    95, 97
  motivation, 117
  plateaus, 139
  at work, 118
  See also exercises; fitness
planning
  meal, 57–58, 62–63, 65
  pregnancy, 190
  in shopping, 107
plasma glucose levels, 37
plateaus, exercise, 139
plate method, 60
pneumonia vaccine, 184
podiatrists, 172, 181
positive self-talk
  as exercise motivator, 138
  as fitness motivator, 117
pramlintide (Symlin), 144, 164
prediabetes, 207
preeclampsia, 194
pregnancy and diabetes, 190–194
pre-mixed insulin, 144
primary doctors, 172
progressive muscle relaxation, 185–186
proteins, 54
puberty, diabetes and, 206

R
race/ethnicity, as risk factor, 17, 18
random blood glucose test, 20
rapid-acting insulin, 146–147
readiness assessment, weight loss, 88–89
recipes, 68–83
  adapting, 106
  carb counting and, 63
  preparation method, changing, 106
  substitutions, 106
relaxation
  breathing, 185
  listen and visualize, 187
  massage, 187–188
  mediation, 187
  progressive muscle, 185–186
  tai chi, 187
  yoga, 187
  See also stress
results, test, 38–39

retinal exam, 179
retinopathy, 28–29
rewards
    healthy eating, 67
    weight loss, 93
risk, 12, 17–18

S

serum creatinine test, 176
serving sizes
    Mayo Clinic Healthy Weight Pyramid and, 97
    reducing, 106
    visual clues, 59
    watching, 58
shoes, 135, 181–182
shopping, smart, 107
short-acting insulin, 146–147
sick days, 215–216
signs and symptoms
    blurred vision, 16
    coronary artery disease, 26
    diabetic ketoacidosis (DKA), 24
    excessive thirst and increased urination, 15
    eye damage (retinopathy), 28–29
    flu-like feeling, 15
    heart attacks, 26–27
    hyperglycemia, 23
    hypoglycemia, 22
    kidney disease (nephropathy), 28
    list of, 15
    nerve damage (neuropathy), 27–28
    red, swollen and tender gums, 16
    slow-healing sores or frequent infections, 16
    stroke, 27
    tingling feet and hands, 16
    type 1 childhood diabetes, 203
    type 2 childhood diabetes, 207
    weight loss or gain, 15–16
silent (asymptomatic) heart attacks, 26
SMART goals
    physical activity, 113
    weight loss, 92–93
smoking, 183
snacks, 104
socks, 180
sores, slow-healing, 16
strengthening exercises, 132–133
stress
    blood glucose and, 46
    healthy ways of dealing with, 110
    individual reactions to, 185
    response, 185
stress management
    four A's, 188
    relaxation, 185–188
    time for yourself and, 188–189
stretching
    benefits of, 131
    do's and don'ts, 130
    exercises, 130–131
    walking and, 124
stroke, 27
substitutions, recipe, 106
sugar
    reducing amount of, 106
    substitutes, 64
sugar-free products, 61
sulfonylureas, 156–157, 158–159
    insulin and, 162–163
    metformin and, 162

TZDs and, 162
    See also oral medications
sweets, 64
syringe
    drawing insulin into, 150
    holding, 151

T

tai chi, 187
taste, changing, 64
teenagers. See childhood diabetes
teeth, caring for, 183
testing
    advanced tools, 36–37
    frequency, 32–34
    performing, 35
    results, recording, 38–39
    results signaling a problem, 46
    See also blood glucose monitoring
tests
    blood and urine, 174
    eye, 179
    fasting blood glucose, 20–21
    glycated hemoglobin (A1C), 20, 174–175
    lipid panel, 175–176
    list of, 177
    oral glucose tolerance, 21
    random blood glucose, 20
    results of, 20
    serum creatinine, 176
    type 1 childhood diabetes, 203–204
    urine, for protein, 176–177
test strips, 33, 41
thiazolidinediones (TZDs), 158–159, 160
    insulin and, 163
    metformin and, 162
    sulfonylurea and, 162
    See also oral medications
thirst, excessive, 15
tingling feet and hands, 16
toenails, 181
total cholesterol, 175
transplant procedures
    islet cell, 168–169
    kidney, 167, 168
    pancreas, 167–168
type 1 childhood diabetes
    goals, 203
    ID tag, 204
    puberty and, 206
    signs and symptoms, 203
    statistics, 201
    testing, 203–204
    treatment, 204–205
    See also childhood diabetes
type 1 diabetes
    as autoimmune disease, 12
    defined, 11–12
    family history and, 12
    illustrated, 14
    insulin injections, 143
    pregnancy and, 192
    process leading to, 12
    risk of developing, 12
    See also diabetes
type 2 childhood diabetes
    increase of, 205–207
    prediabetes, 207
    screening, 207
    signs and symptoms, 207

statistics, 201
    treatment, 207
    See also childhood diabetes
type 2 diabetes
    defined, 13
    healthy weight and, 85–86
    herbal remedies and, 157
    illustrated, 14
    insulin and, 163
    insulin dependence and, 13
    as national epidemic, 11
    oral medications, 156–161
    pregnancy and, 192
    risk factors, 85
    risk of developing, 12
    statistics, 9, 11
    See also diabetes
TZDs. See thiazolidinediones

U

urination, frequent, 15
urine test, 176–177

V

vaccinations, 184

W

waist circumference, 87
walking, 124–125
    See also aerobic exercise
warming up, 135
water
    energy density and, 98
    need for, 128
weight
    checking, 173
    loss or gain as symptom, 15–16
    as risk factor, 17
weight loss
    barriers, action guide for, 90–91
    calorie goal, 96
    challenge of, 86
    eating triggers and, 103
    energy density and, 98–100
    first steps toward, 94
    getting back on track, 109–110
    goals, 92–93
    habits for a lifetime, 110
    meal routine and, 104–105
    need determination for, 86–88
    readiness assessment, 88–91
    setbacks, overcoming, 109–111
    smart shopping and, 107
    tools for goal evaluation, 111
    willpower vs. self-control and, 108
    See also healthy weight
weight training, 133
well-being, fitness and, 115
willpower vs. self-control, 108
women's health
    menopause, 195–196
    menstruation, 195
    pregnancy, 190–194
work, physical activity at, 118

Y

yoga, 187

Visit our online store

for a wide selection of books, newsletters and DVDs developed by Mayo Clinic doctors and editorial staff.

Discover practical, easy-to-understand information on topics of interest to millions of health-conscious people like you …

➤ *Mayo Clinic Health Letter* — our award-winning monthly newsletter filled with practical information on today's health and medical news

➤ *Mayo Clinic Family Health Book* — the ultimate home health reference

➤ *The Mayo Clinic Diet: Eat Well, Enjoy Life, Lose Weight* — step-by-step guidance from Mayo Clinic weight-loss experts to help you achieve a healthy weight.

➤ *Mayo Clinic Book of Alternative Medicine* — the new approach to combining the best of natural therapies and conventional medicine

➤ *Mayo Clinic Book of Home Remedies* — discover how to prevent, treat or manage over 120 common health conditions at home

➤ *Mayo Clinic on Digestive Health* — learn how to identify and treat digestive problems before they become difficult to manage

➤ *Plus* — books on arthritis, aging, diabetes, high blood pressure and other conditions

Mayo Clinic brings you more of the health information you're looking for!

www.Store.MayoClinic.com